No Stress

at the Speed of

THOUGHT

MyStress
Reset Kit©

RITA PERSAUD-KONG

Dedication

*In Memory of my beloved parents, who
taught me the Yoga way of life*

Disclaimer

This book in no way seeks to give medical advice, treat, diagnose, or prescribe. The information herein contained is not a substitute for consultation with a licensed physician and health care provider.

Contents

Preface

I have practiced Yoga for over thirty years. When I first had the idea of writing this book, it was simply to share with everyone my stress reset tools and techniques, which have worked for me so well through the years. I thought that if it helped only a few people I would have made a contribution in this regard and it seemed like a simple idea. However, in trying to put my stress reset tools and techniques into a conceptual framework I was forced to ask why and how it worked for me. The answer was quite mind boggling, in that science does not fully recognize much less define the concepts of the mind and consciousness. Even how the body is kept in balance is not precisely understood. While there is a plethora of literature on the body-mind connection, it remains an elusive concept and so much about our brain is not yet known. Notwithstanding, since no one seems to have all the answers, I hope that what works for me will work for you. You just need to have an open mind.

PART I: ALL ABOUT YOUR THOUGHTS

The challenge is to obtain peace, calm and stillness of thought in a complex, often chaotic and conflicted world.

Introduction

Every day our body and mind is subjected to various demands. It is busy from the moment we get up in the morning to the moment we go to bed at night and can't sleep, tossing and turning, replaying in our mind's eye the situations we perceived as difficult, the events that caused us to worry, the problems we could not solve, the conflict we could not resolve and the decisions we find so difficult to make, thoughts and more thoughts.

Indeed, as we close our eyes and try to sleep, chaotic thoughts parade through our mind and sleep eludes us. Stress begins to take its toll surreptitiously on our body and mind. We could go on day in and day out without realizing we have stress, until it becomes chronic and starts to affect our health. This book seeks to provide you with lifestyle tools and techniques to avoid stress by the way you think about and handle situations and events in your life. Additionally, where you cannot avoid the effects of stress, you must try to reverse these effects or learn to manage and live with them while achieving a calm state of mind and body. In short, these lifestyle tools and techniques allow you to reset your body and mind to achieve inner and outer harmony.

Have you ever noticed how some people are rarely affected by stress, how they remain cool, calm and collected in the midst of chaos, adversity and catastrophe? Yet others get violent, quarrel, cry and are overwhelmed by stress. Why can some people control their thoughts and cope while others cannot?

Anxiety, anger and violence start during early learning. Children who are learning to think and don't know how to solve a problem turn to aggression. Observe the children who are likely to become violent teens; they solve their problems physically. A child wants a toy that another child has, so he grabs it and then pushes the other child. A fight ensues. The teacher or the parent disciplines him by either scolding or beating and this causes stress to all concerned.

The distinction is often made between managing stress and managing life. The person who copes manages life and the person who cannot cope needs to manage stress. Can you visualize a person's normal state as that of peace, joy and positivity and his abnormal state as that of anger, depression and negativity? We learn to cope and manage life, including the way we think, act and feel, in early childhood. Much of what causes stress is negative thinking that became a habit when we were children.

For example if you scold a child to get him to do his homework, your negative attitude creates stress and does not achieve the results you want. So if you do not scold but ask the child in a peaceful manner to do his work, the child will respond and do his work peacefully. But what if the child does not respond to a peaceful request? Then how will anger and scolding help? Instead of blaming and scolding the child, show compassion and understanding and help the child define the problem facing him. For example, ask why he does not want to do his homework.

Once the problem is defined, there is no need to scold but only to help the child to find solutions to the problem. In other words, replace negative energy flows with positive energy flows. For example, a child having difficulty learning to write was scolded repeatedly, resulting in tantrums and tears. When asked why he could not write, he said that the pencil was falling out of his hand. So this problem was fixed by teaching him the proper grip. But then there was another problem: his writing was not in a straight line. It turned out that he was not focusing. So the child was taught to direct his attention to the point where the pencil should touch the paper. He was also taught to meditate. After some practice, he learned to write without stress. In such cases, positive energy flows and creates peace and calm. Over time and with repeated problem solving, the child got into the habit and mental state of remaining calm in difficult situations while his mind sought solutions.

Most of us spend our entire lives, from early childhood to going to school to working to meeting family responsibilities and commitments, barely having time for ourselves. When we are in a stressful situation, most of us do not accept that we are stressed. Why? Because to do so, especially in a work environment, we believe, is to admit that we cannot cope which is a no-no on so many levels.

Do we consider who we are, as a human body and how our body works? If we knew it from high school biology, is it uppermost in our minds as we go about our daily living? For example, when we see a cinnamon roll, an apple or a bar of chocolate, what comes to mind is "Yummy taste" or "This smells delicious." Not a thought comes to mind about what happens to the food after it is eaten. Perhaps if it did, we would be able to focus on what we eat, how much we eat and when we eat, all of which would go a long way in ensuring a healthy life.

Come with me on an exploration of stress and its effect on our well-being, including what our body is comprised of and how it works. Learn about the basics of homeostasis and how it keeps the body in equilibrium. Why it is necessary to keep our body in balance? Does your mind exist in your brain? Or is it separate and apart? Or does it exist at all? This does not matter, because the mind still affects our bodily functions and stress.

How aware are you of your conscious thoughts? Are decisions made by your conscious or subconscious mind? How do you perceive stress? Is a stressor a stress because we think it is? We will consider the incredible power of thoughts and how our well-being is guided by our thoughts.

PART II:
NATURE'S MARVEL

We are nature's most complex creation:
the conscious body and mind.

Body

The *Oxford Dictionary* defines the body as "the whole physical structure of a person" But how well do you know your body? The physical structure yes because we look into the mirror and there we are, but wish that we could also see the internal structure and workings of our body in the mirror. The physical body and its internal structures, for which science, technology and medicine can diagnose illnesses and prescribe remedies, are unfortunately not visible to us. We cannot see the internal structure of our own body in real-time, just as we cannot see the quantum micro world. These are the stuff that science fiction is made of, but maybe in the future this technology will become available to us. Understanding the dynamics and maintaining health and wellness of our body is a complicated process and is a challenge to each one of us as we go through our daily lives. The World Health Organization has defined health as "a state of complete physical, mental, and social well-being and not merely the absence of disease or infirmity."

Human biology is the scientific study of the body that looks at the structure and how our body functions on the level of cells, tissues, organs and systems. How the body evolved and hereditary factors are known as genetics and are key to understanding how the body works.

Chemistry is the branch of science that deals with the identification of the substances of which matter is composed; it is an investigation of their properties, the way they interact, and the way atoms form molecules. Biochemistry looks at how carbohydrates, fats, proteins, hormones, enzymes and other chemicals work in our body.

Physics is the branch of science concerned with the nature and properties of energy and matter. It includes the studies of electricity, light and magnetism. The relevance of physics to our body is perhaps less obvious, though it is very important.

With respect to our body and mind, these disciplines and the many different fields that these disciplines are subdivided into seem to be independent of each other. Connecting the dots seems a distant goal. For example, even the names given to stress hormones differ according to the discipline that is referring to it. Whatever the reason for these developments, they are certainly not beneficial from the perceptive of the layperson trying to understand the working of his body.

Mind

We have a mind and body, but do we understand the intricacies of how they work? The *Oxford Dictionary* defines *mind* as the element of a person that enables them to be aware of the world and their experiences, to think and to feel. Some popular usages indicative of our mind being the same as our thoughts are "in our mind," the things we see in our "mind's eye" as a result of which we "make up our mind" or "change our mind," or we can't decide about something and are of "two minds." So the bottom line is that only we can know "our own mind". Others could only interpret what we consciously or subconsciously communicate to them.

Our thoughts, feelings, sensations, learning, memory, responses and other functions are possible through the fascinating communication process between the nerve cells of our brain, called neurons and our nervous system. Through stimulus, neurons receive information about our internal and the external environment, communicate this information and coordinate appropriate responses. The neurons in our brain communicate when two neurons connect at a space called the synapse, where the neurons "touch" and send messages through electrochemical activity. Specific thoughts are produced by specific neuron firing patterns when cells communicate with one another. So thinking enables cells to communicate with each other and when cells communicate with each other, we think. A question arises: do neuron firings cause us to think or when we think neuron firings are caused? We will look at this question again when we examine the stress response.

So the brain facilitates and enables the mind to think, even if it is not clear to science exactly why and how. Science is uncertain as to whether or not the mind exists. One view is that the mind emerges from the physical connections between neurons and is therefore an emergent property of the brain. Another view is that the mind is the activities of the brain. Yet another view is that the mind is not the brain but it is energy.

Our legal systems are predicated on our being of body, mind, intention and conscious awareness. The law recognizes the mind, the concept of free will and our responsibility for our actions. The Rule of Law and Order is predicated on the core principle of truth. Guilt or innocence in a court of law is determined by a judge and or a jury. A fundamental principle of Criminal Law is that both the physical act itself and the intention to commit the act must be present to constitute a crime. Sir Edward Coke made a classic statement of the Common Law: *actus non facit reum nisi mens sit rea,* which is Latin for "the act does not make a person guilty, unless their mind is also guilty." Legislation in both Criminal Law and Civil Law have used specific words to indicate a guilty mind, such as *intentionally, knowingly, recklessly, maliciously, negligently* and *fraudulently.* So the law recognizes and embraces the mind-body connection.

Neuroscience seems to be leading in the direction of determinism, the idea that our brain works in a predetermined way and that ultimately we may become some kind of machine not responsible for our actions and not having free will. If it turns out that this is so, then it would severely impact our legal and judicial systems. But we can take heart in the fact that criminals and wrongdoers will not escape punishment. Whether we are machines or not, we must live in society (even if it's a society of machines) and there must be rules and laws in society, making punishment a consequence of our actions in order to prevent chaos. Legal systems will adopt and evolve.

The current neuroscientific view appears to be that, while the neuron circuitry of the brain and its overall connectivity patterns are under genetic control (genes), stimuli from the environment, our experiences and our training affect neuron connectivity and growth. Genes alone cannot provide the complete picture, because while genes are fixed from the moment of conception, our brain's neural circuitry changes throughout life. Neurons adjust by strengthening or weakening their connections; they create and eliminate synapses and they grow and rewire. As a consequence, everyone's brain is unique in terms of at least its neuron connectivity and the emergent thought.

Neuroscience needs to demystify the brain and develop a connectome. *Connectome* is a scientific term that means a comprehensive understanding and mapping of the organization of neural interactions, activity and connectivity of how the process or set of rules and algorithms governing our human brain and our thoughts work. Only then can some of these fundamental questions be definitively answered.

According to the Honda Research Institute, its brain machine interface will enable people to control robots using their mind and thought power. It may well be that in the future our feelings and emotions will distinguish us from machines, but we will be able to measure stress accurately and maybe stress reset will be a synch. Further, with scientific understanding of all the intricate workings of the brain, its connection with the mind and consciousness should become clear.

Maybe we are wired and encoded to function like a computer, but it may not yield the answer to who we are. Why? Because while science reductionist methods that is, breaking things down to its finest to understand how it works, will explain how and why all the nerve circuits and connectome work, it may not explain the connection between the physical nerve cell and the abstract thought. More importantly, it may not explain how the thought originated or emerged. This may be where our soul, spirit, and God step in.

Mind-Body

Plato, Aristotle, Descartes, Spinoza and so many other philosophers considered the body-mind connection and came up with monism and its various forms as well as dualism and its various forms. These hypotheses have inspired much debate through the centuries, but there has been no resolution to the problem. In the seventeenth century, the philosopher Rene Descartes reasoned that the mind is not physical, because physical things like the body occupy space, are spatial, and are measurable. The mind cannot be measured and though mental activity occurs in time, it does not occupy space and has a free will. Descartes's ideas that the mind is nonphysical and that there is a divide between it and the physical world was called mind-body dualism and became known as the mind-body problem.

The ancient seers (rishis or sages) of India founded Ayurveda, India's natural medicine system based on beliefs contained in the Vedas, text written in Sanskrit. According to Ayurveda, the body, mind, and consciousness are all parts of the whole and influence each other in the working of the body and mind. Certainly the Common Law seems to agree with this ancient Indian view regarding the mind and body being one.

Does the mind have to be a part of the brain to be justifiably a part of the body? Science is concerned with the physical form, not so much with the mental form. Yet health for everyone is being in a condition of wellness on every level the physical, mental and emotional, even if we don't understand precisely how this is achieved. Body and mind translated from an individual point of view is definitely not a problem. So we don't consider that there is a problem with our body and our mind being the same or separate from each other. You might think, *well, at least if we don't understand, the scientists and physicians do, so we are safe.* This is true if you are ill and have a disease, then medicine can identify and diagnose what is wrong and prescribe a remedy. But medicine generally cannot tell you why it went wrong or how to avoid or prevent it.

Consciousness

Understanding how stress affects our body and mind, observing our body structure, physical appearances, comforts, discomforts, pain, thoughts, feelings, sensations and perceptions are all critical factors in our ability to cope with stress. Numerous theories regarding the nature of consciousness have evolved from the beginning of time. How then do we explain consciousness? Some believe that consciousness is not a valid concept because it is incoherent and illusory. Others believe that the individual conscious mind is part of a whole, the universal conscious mind that resides in God, Brahma, or whatever divine being.

Science has hesitated to give recognition to the term *consciousness* and then there are the terms *preconscious*, *unconscious* and *subconscious*, which are recognized in psychology and made famous by psychologists Sigmund Freud, Carl Jung and others. But, again the views and theories are divergent. Consciousness is a challenge yet to be resolved.

Neural correlates of consciousness studies use brain imaging techniques to examine the relationship between a person's thoughts and the simultaneous neural process activities taking place in their brain. These studies anticipate that a pattern will emerge that explains consciousness. So far neuroscientist and neurobiologist have learned much about the brain processes, but no single theory has emerged giving a complete understanding about consciousness. Other models for explaining consciousness have gone beyond neural activities of the brain, placing consciousness at the fundamental level of Quantum Mechanics.

Quantum Mechanics suggests that microparticles behave in strange ways, completely unlike anything we see in our everyday lives. At this time, it shows that our observations of the laws of nature through measurement produce probabilistic outcomes: microparticles occupy many states at the same time. Closely connected microparticles when separated remain interconnected instantaneously and microparticles can pass through solid objects. Quantum Mechanics tells us how some things are possible and probable but not certain. Indeed, the strange things can be explained only by complex mathematics. It is an unfolding story and therefore the interpretations with respect to consciousness are numerous. However we are no closer to a universal understanding of the nature of consciousness.

Ordinary Meanings

So again I resort to the Oxford Dictionary, which defines *consciousness* as "the state of being aware of and responsive to one's surroundings." *Unconscious* is defined first as "the state of being unconscious: someone gave me a crack across the head and I slipped into unconsciousness" and "the state of being uniformed or unaware: part of her beauty was her unconsciousness of it." Subconscious is defined as "concerning the part of the mind of which one is not fully aware but which influences one's actions and feelings: my subconscious fear." The Oxford Dictionary also notes that the word *subconscious* is not in technical use in psychoanalysis, where *unconscious* is preferred. In this book, the term *subconscious* is used because it has only one meaning and therefore is not subject to ambiguity.

Is It Conscious or Subconscious?

In the 1970s, Benjamin Libet et al. found through experiments that subconscious processes in the brain are the true initiators of our actions and that a signal called the "readiness-potential" occurred before a conscious decision is taken. Building on this research, in 2011 Stefan Bode et al. used functional Magnetic Resonance Imaging (fMRI) to demonstrate that the brain activity showed that decisions are subconsciously prepared several seconds ahead of time about how a person is going to decide. But the research did not investigate when the final decision is made or whether a decision prepared subconsciously can be reversed by the conscious mind.

It must seem obvious to us that we have free will when we just made a decision to eat ice cream, but some philosophers and now neuroscientists say that we may be wrong. Our choice was predetermined because it was the outcome of our experience, because it was random, or because it was determined by our subconscious state before our conscious took the decision.

What has this got to do with stress? Well, most of my lifestyle tools and techniques to avoid and relieve stress are based on our free will, our thoughts, our beliefs and our ability to make decisions and choices. However, if it's all predetermined, we cannot make choices, develop a stress reset plan and by extension live a healthy life.

With regard to our body and mind, free will is not doing what we want to do without regard for the law and nature. Additionally, determinism should not mean that everything is predetermined. First, we are sentient that is, we are able to perceive and feel things and we have a conscience. Second, our actions are partly conscious and partly subconscious through the activities of the voluntary and the involuntary organ systems of our body. The debate between free will and determinism seems pointless as we are blessed with both the conscious and the subconscious and therefore there is varying degree of free will and determinism within each of us. In the final analysis, we make the decision to eat ice cream whether the decision was made by our conscious or subconscious mind.

Consciousness defines our existence and reality and it is awareness of a portion of our mind and brain activities. Our subconscious makes up most of the rest of our brain activity and its content. Our subconscious state influences our perceptions, thoughts, feelings and behaviors. We can become aware of our subconscious mental content through the focus of our attention or mindfulness.

Science, philosophy, psychology, neuroscience, religion, law and other disciplines all have different views of the mind, consciousness-brain and body connection. It is amazing that something that each one of us has and that we can intuitively explain is inexplicable to the finest minds. In fact, at any given point most of us are unaware of our mind, our thoughts and in particular our brain activities even though these activities influence the way we perceive things, the way we think, our feelings, our motivations, our behaviors and our actions. However, I believe that consciousness or awareness can be cultivated and become a tool we use to develop and enhance the thought processes and activities of the mind to our best advantage.

When we learn to walk as a toddler, ride a bike as a child, or drive a car as a teenager, the processes are the same. A group of neurons communicate with each other. At the beginning, because the neurons have not communicated before about these activities (the neurons are also learning) you stumbled while trying to walk or you lost your balance and fell off the bike or you pressed the accelerator when you should have pressed the brakes. This is a conscious process as you learn and try to perfect the activity. After a while though, our neurons communicate, learn and imprint the process so you can walk, ride a bike and drive a car. Eventually, we perform these activities mostly subconsciously. Fundamentally, everything we do works like this. Our thoughts are powerful and amazing. What we think determines how we perform, who we become and how well we maintain our body wellness.

The well-being of our body and mind appears to be a state that emerges from the interaction of our mind and brain. Such interactions are characterized by all our experiences on the personal and social levels, producing our awareness and conscious reality, even though we don't know how it all works. For the purpose of this book, we will adopt what may be considered by some as a simplistic view that the mind, consciousness, brain and body are parts of a whole, one entity and that each part can and does work in tandem to keep our body in balance.

Perception

Perception is where stress begins or not, because perception brings conscious awareness, informs our mind thoughts and connects our mind and body. Perception is a process that allows us to experience through awareness everything around us by way of our senses. Our senses are therefore critical to the way we perceive things and our response to such perception determines whether we are stressed or not. We perceive by our various sensory systems that is, seeing with our eyes, smelling with our nose, hearing with our ears, feeling with our skin and tasting with our tongue. At any given time, there is a huge amount of stimulation bombarding our senses, but not all stimuli reach our conscious awareness.

There is more to light than we can see, because the colors we see are only some wavelengths of light. There are several other wavelengths that together make up electromagnetic radiation (light). The electromagnetic (EM) spectrum ranks radiation from lowest energy with longest wavelengths to highest energy with shortest wavelengths. The higher the energy, the more dangerous the radiation is. Light is described by numbers called frequencies. As the number gets higher on the EM spectrum, the light goes from red to blue to violet to ultraviolet to X-rays to gamma rays. On the other end of the EM spectrum, the frequency gets lower. The light goes from blue to red to infrared, such as heat waves, microwaves, television waves, and radio waves. But we could see only up to violet.

The activities of our body are coordinated by and rely on the input of information from stimuli received from our internal and external environments. A stimulus is detected by sensory receptors. The simplest sensory receptor is a neuron, which can detect a stimulus and transform it to a nerve impulse. The complex receptors are the sense organs, such as the eyes and ears. Exteroceptor signals reach our body from the outside environment and most are located on our skin or in our eyes and our ears. Proprioceptor signals originate from within our body from our muscular and skeletal systems. Interoceptor signals arise from the internal organs, such as our heart, our lungs and our intestines. They are mostly processed at the subconscious level. Exteroceptor signals and the proprioceptor signals are mostly processed at the conscious level and are subjective sensory experiences in the sense that we feel cold or we feel warm or we feel pain.

Our sensory receptors detect several types of stimuli and encode and transform those stimuli into electrical nerve impulses that then propagate from neuron to neuron through our central nervous system, in which they are decoded to provide the required response. A photoreceptor detects electromagnetic radiation from light stimuli received through our eyes and transforms and encodes it to a nerve impulse. We are told it takes only five or six photons of light to activate a nerve impulse and send a message to our brain. An electroreceptor detects electromagnetic energy from electrical stimuli received and transforms and encodes it into a nerve impulse. A mechanoreceptor detects mechanical energy through sound from hearing, through touch from feeling, and through pressure on the body and transforms and encodes it into a nerve impulse. A thermoreceptor detects thermal energy from change in our body temperature and transforms and encodes it into a nerve impulse. A chemoreceptor detects chemical energy through humidity, smell and taste and transforms and encodes it into a nerve impulse.

The task of all these sensory receptors is to translate the stimulus to electrical signals in the form of an action potential called a nerve impulse (*action potential* and *nerve impulse* are used interchangeably). In a sensory receptor, a nerve impulse arises near the terminal branches. The process is similar to synaptic activation with voltage-gated channels described in Part III below. To this extent, the transmission of a stimulus to sensory receptors is only partly known.

The process by which sensory receptors transform a stimulus into a nerve impulse is called transduction and there is a lack of clarity as to precisely how this is done. We are told that transduction is a process in which our sensory systems encode stimulus energy as neural messages that our brain can interpret. Sensory receptors are known as biological transducers. So, for example, our eyes convert light energy, which is a very thin bandwidth from the EM spectrum. The beautiful colors and hues we see and everything in the world around us depends upon the light frequency and wavelength, which somehow informs the perception from which our thoughts emerge.

So stimulus is transmitted by transduction. Sensation, feeling, thought and perception originate and are encoded into nerve impulses that are propagated via nerve cells to the central nervous system and the brain, where evaluation is done to produce sensation, feeling, thought and perception. However, a question arises as to where and how these sensation, feeling, thought and perception have emerged. Is it at the sensory receptors, the propagation process through the nervous system or is it in the brain. The answer is not entirely clear, as neuroscience and the endless fields of science are not sure. Perception seems effortless because we are not aware that these complex processes are taking place. Most of us would say, "What do you mean, it isn't clear where my thoughts come from? Of course they come from my mind." Others would say, "My thoughts are from my brain," and yet others would say, "They are from my sensory receptors."

Whether sensation, thought, and perception emerge from the mind or the body or from both, they adversely impact stress. So senses are from the realm of the mind to the physical world and vice versa. Intuition, understanding, insight, and becoming aware of external stimuli are keys to our ability to perceive. Perception is critical in decision making and taking action, because the meaning we give to a stimulus we receive informs our choices. Everyone's perception is different, because our perception is influenced by the transduction process, our memory of the past, our expectation and prediction of the future and our beliefs.

It is believed that the neurons firing in our nervous system and our brain cause our conscious and our subconscious to analyze and interpret that which is perceived. Therefore, the same thing can be perceived differently by different persons and our perception is not necessarily the reality or as some would say, we create our own reality. Our brain and our mind perceive and determine our responses accordingly. So we have a choice when faced with a potentially stressful situation through our awareness, perception, belief and ultimately our thoughts. We can choose to respond or not to respond. So our thoughts determine whether there is stress or no stress.

Our perception alters our reality. To change our behavior, we must change what we believe and our thoughts. Our subconscious works on thoughts that are dominating our conscious mind. The degree of power we put in our conscious thoughts will reflect in our subconscious thought and a powerful conscious thought will cause a powerful subconscious thought.

So, become aware of your conscious thoughts and beliefs, because your subconscious will adopt them and believe them, whether they are true or not. For example, you believe that you can't stop eating chocolate, and you generate a conscious thought: "I can't stop eating chocolate." Your brain will not question this belief; its neurons will come together and connect and you will find that you really can't stop eating chocolate. This belief would come about because you tried to stop without success. So, stop the conscious thinking and rewire the program and connectivity of your neurons. How is this done? Through Vipassana, also known as Insight Meditation, this harnesses the power of your subconscious mind to make changes in your behavior that you find difficult to make by your conscious will-power.

In this book the mind is considered to be our thoughts in the realm of our awareness, perception and beliefs. Consciousness is the acute awareness of the activities of our mind. How conscious or aware we are of all the activities of our mind depends on each individual's perception and belief, which are subjective, different and unique to each of us. Each individual mind has a nature, awareness, perception and belief of its own. It is subtle and can be volatile and our ability to control our thoughts brings peace while our inability to control our thoughts brings stress and is responsible for illnesses. So stress and our wellness depend on the speed of our thoughts and our ability to control those thoughts.

PART III:
THE UNIVERSE
WITHIN

Our body's processes, its all-natural automation, are designed to self-regulate and heal.

Stress

Stress is one of the major factors that can cause imbalances and prevent our body from functioning properly and maintaining balance. Physician Hans Selye coined the term *stress* and defined it as "the nonspecific response of the body to any demands whether it is caused by, or results in, pleasant or unpleasant conditions." He drew a distinction between *distress* and *eustress*. *Eustress* is Greek for good stress, when stress is quickly resolved. *Distress* is bad stress, when stress is excessive and prolonged.

Both distress and eustress result in the activation of what Selye termed the General Adaptation Syndrome (GAS), which he wrote about in 1936. He identified GAS as having three stages of adaptation: Alarm Reaction, Resistance and Exhaustion. The first, the Alarm Reaction Stage, is one in which a threat or a stressor is identified and the fight-or-flight response is triggered. The second, the Resistance Stage, is when we adjust to the stress and our body begins to adapt the demands, but the body cannot keep up its adaptation indefinitely. The third, the Exhaustion Stage, is when there is a "burnout" because the stress is prolonged, the adaption process is exhausted and our body is unable to regain normal function and balance. Long-term chronic stress leads to disease and illnesses such as ulcer, high blood pressure, diabetes, cardiovascular disease and digestive systems malfunctions.

Many other researchers have proposed other definitions of stress, and researchers now focus on behavioral and cognitive causes, so stress is viewed by some as a mind-body phenomenon. While most experts generally agree with Selye's definition of stress, it is difficult to find a definition acceptable to all scientists, physicians, psychologists, the general public and others. Indeed, the general public tends to use the term *stress* in different ways such as having too much responsibilities and pressures. We use the term *stressed out* to describe when we feel overloaded and overwhelmed by everything and our inability to cope with the pressures of daily living.

"Stress is difficult for scientists to define because it is a subjective sensation associated with varied symptoms that differ for each of us," said Dr. Paul J. Rosch, president of the American Institute of Stress. The Oxford Dictionary defines *stress* as "a state of affair involving demand on physical or mental energy." In this book, *stress* is considered to be the response of the mind and body to any demand place upon it. This definition puts the emphasis on our response to the demand and not on the demand itself. The response can be good or bad. It depends on the capacity of our body and mind to respond well or not to respond and result in stress. The demand could be both physiological (physical or body) and psychological (mental or mind). Usually, physical stress cannot be avoided, such as being startled by a sudden loud noise, being injured in an accident or having surgery. However, we have the ability to avoid mental stress.

Homeostasis

In 1857 the French physiologist Claude Bernard advanced the idea *"la fixité du milieu interieur est la condition d'une vie libre et independante,"* which is French for "the constancy of the internal environment is the condition for a free and independent life." He described it as the principles of dynamic equilibrium, a steady state in the internal bodily environment necessary for survival, a balance that external changes in the environment can alter. Dynamic equilibrium was termed *homeostasis* by the American physiologist Walter B. Cannon in his 1932 book, *The Wisdom of the Body.* He advanced the homeostasis model, the idea that our body's internal processes maintain equilibrium and wellness. *Homeostasis* is Greek for "staying the same."

Another model, called *allostasis,* was advanced by Sterling and Eyer in 1988. Homeostasis emphasizes the states and optimal set points for equilibrium, while allostasis emphasizes the optimal operating ranges for equilibrium. Some have argued that allostasis is no more than a renaming of the original concept of homeostasis. Others believe it has not added to the homeostasis model in bringing clarity to the understanding of our body's internal processes regarding stress. Yet others have advanced the concept of "stress neurocircuitry" on the basis that stress, as an integral part of the homeostasis and allostasis models, detracts from the development of a conceptual framework that allows for dealing with stress. In this book I refer to the body's dynamic equilibrium as homeostasis.

Stress and homeostasis are at different ends of the body spectrum and they work to tell the story of our lives from the inside out. Stress makes us susceptible to illnesses and diseases, while homeostasis keeps our body in a dynamic balance and maintains good health and wellness. Here is how: Homeostasis is achieved when our body maintains a stable internal environment in response to fluctuation and change. If there were no balance in our internal environment, our cells, tissues, organs, systems, enzymes and hormones would not work properly and we would be susceptible to diseases and illnesses. One of the major factors affecting this balance is stress, but before we consider how stress affects homeostasis, let's look at how homeostasis works.

The homeostasis model is based on the concept that there are mechanisms and processes regulating our internal organs and bodily systems and working in tandem, as a whole, to contribute to the maintenance of homoeostasis. Homeostatic regulation involves the working of negative feedback loop and positive feedback loop mechanisms through the receptors (sensors), the control (command center) and the effectors. When there is a change in the internal or external environment, the negative feedback or the positive feedback is triggered.

A sensory receptor receives stimulus when there is a change in the environment, using nerve pathways to send messages to the command center. Most often it is the brain that receives the information, processes it, and decides what set point value should be maintained in the body. The command center then sends electrical signals along nerves to effectors, which, depending on the information received, oppose or enhance the stimulus to correct any deviation caused by the changed environment. This brings the body back to normal set point and reestablishes homeostasis. For example, when there is a temperature change, the sensory receptor in the skin and the hypothalamus sense the change and the brain sends a command to affect a response to decrease or increase our body temperature to achieve a balance.

To achieve and keep homeostasis, the body must limit fluctuations and reset imbalances and it uses the negative feedback mechanism to do this. Negative feedback is similar to the operations of an air-conditioner that automatically switches off when the thermostat senses that the temperature is higher than the set normal point or switches on when the temperature is lower than the set normal point. This switch off and switch on is the negative feedback that allows the temperature to maintain its normal set point.

A positive feedback response is the reverse of a negative feedback, because it amplifies the change in the environment (the thermostat ceases to work), and this causes a homeostatic imbalance. Positive feedback is less frequent and can be both harmful and beneficial. It is beneficial in the case of the secretion of the hormone oxytocin, which stimulates muscular contractions of the uterus during childbirth. It can be harmful in the case of heart failure, when the negative feedback mechanism becomes overwhelmed and destructive positive feedback mechanisms take over to result in heart failure.

Homeostasis reaches from the cells to the organs and systems of our body to maintain a constant internal body environment. Several key homeostatic controls are essential to life namely the regulation of temperature, water levels, and glucose concentration and the removal of urea and carbon dioxide. To understand how stress affects homeostasis, the following is a brief overview of our cells and organ systems, highly complex and dynamic processes that assist in the maintenance of homeostasis.

Body Cells

Our body cells comprise a nucleus, which controls the cell activities, genes, cytoplasm, mitochondria and other organelles, which are surrounded by the cell membrane. Basic cell processes are protein synthesis and energy production. Our cells work together, each carrying out its own function with all that the cell needs to survive, such as oxygen and nutrients. The normal balance of our internal state depends on our adaptation to stimuli. In this regard, the main part of our cell that works to maintain homeostasis is the cell membrane. This is the outer wall of the cell that separates the cell from the outer world. Basically, it protects the cell's homeostasis from disruptive stimuli.

Body Energy

Energy can be defined as the capacity to do work. For our body to keep working, it requires a continuous supply of energy. According to the laws of thermodynamics, energy can neither be created nor destroyed, but it can be transferred from one form to another. This occurs in various forms, such as light, chemical, heat, electrical, mechanical and sound. A good example is striking a match, when the chemical energy in the match head is transferred to heat, light and sound. Energy is used in many ways to keep our body in homeostasis and in particular energy is used in the electrical transmission of nerve impulses.

Our cells are made up of atoms, which are made up of protons that have a positive charge, neutrons that have a neutral charge and electrons that have a negative charge. When these charges are out of balance, an atom becomes either negatively or positively charged and this allows electrons to flow from one atom to another. This flow of electron or negative charge is called electricity. Theoretically, our body generates electricity through its huge mass of atoms and this also facilitates communication between cells, organs and body systems. We are our own "power grid."

Energy in a cell is in the form of molecules called adenosine triphosphate (ATP), which supply the cell with energy for cellular activity. For a muscle cell, this would be muscle contractions and for an immune cell, it would be killing bacterial invaders. ATP is the energy found throughout our body and is used to generate electrical impulses in the nerves and to power our photoreceptors, electroreceptors, mechanoreceptors and thermoreceptors, all of which send nerve impulses to our brain and enable perception.

We get energy from the food we eat. Food is metabolized or broken down to make energy. Metabolism is the physical and chemical changes taking place in our body. It converts the energy in food, mainly fatty acids and sugar, to energy in our cells for the use of cell activities. The key part of this metabolic process takes place in the mitochondria, sometimes referred to as the "cellular power plant," which exist in each of our cells. Our body requires a normal amount of ATP to be stored and constantly recycled every day. The more active our body becomes, the more ATP is needed and the mitochondria constantly produce ATP. ATP is released as needed by the splitting of the ATP molecule into adenosine diphospate (ADP) and inorganic phosphorus. ATP production is done by the process of cell respiration, which uses oxygen to generate energy. One of the benefits of doing aerobic exercise is that it provides greater oxygen intake, which in turn enables rapid production of ATP. We breathe in air, which has an oxygen content of approximately 21 percent.

Cell Respiration

Cell respiration (as distinct from body respiration of breathing) is the process by which chemical energy in organic molecules is released by oxidation and this energy is available in our body in the form of ATP. If this process requires oxygen, it is called aerobic respiration. If it takes place in the absence of oxygen, it is called anaerobic respiration. The organic chemicals most commonly used are carbohydrates, glucose and fats, which are broken down by a series of enzyme-controlled reactions to release a small amount of energy, some of which is transferred to molecules called ATP.

ATP is the energy carrier of cells, which use it as necessary. ATP is therefore referred to as the "universal energy carrier" or "energy currency" and the battery is often used as an analogy. From a battery you could get light, mechanical, sound and electrical energy. The convenience of a battery is that the same source of energy can be used to perform a wide range of work and this is the same for ATP. Another analogy is that, like some batteries, ATP is rechargeable. Energy is used in a factory to make the battery and so too ATP is made using energy from the oxidation of organic molecules during respiration.

The ATP production process, whether from glucose or fatty acids, comes with an adverse effect, namely the production of free radicals, which can damage the mitochondria's DNA, deoxyribonucleic acid. DNA is a self-replicating material present in all cells as the main constituent of chromosomes and it carries genetic information. The good news is that when properly working, the mitochondria can deal with the free radicals through the natural production of glutathione, an antioxidant. However this process slows down as we age.

Mitochondria do their hardest work inside our brain, which uses a large amount of energy and oxygen. If the mitochondria in the brain are unable to produce ATP, the mitochondria in the other parts of the body are unable to share their ATP due to the blood brain barrier. So it is critical for the mitochondria in our brain to function efficiently.

Adaptation Energy

According to Selye, we have hidden adaptation energy in the body that it uses up during stress. When all the adaptation energy is used up, this leads to exhaustion and death follows. Further, each of us inherits a certain amount of adaptation energy and the amount is determined by our genetic makeup. So we can draw upon this energy thriftily for a long, stress-free, uneventful and simple life or we can spend all the energy on a stressful, intense and exiting life, which may be shorter, as there is just so much adaptation energy to be used and no more. If this is correct, the question arises as to how individuals can manage this store of limited adaptation energy through a long life? The answer, of course, may be to live a relatively stress-free life.

Studies have shown that ATP production peaks at age twenty and as we grow older, our cells' ability to produce ATP gradually declines and so does our energy levels. Stress, an unhealthy life-style and disease contribute to this decline. Another factor is the production of oxidants or free radicals, which studies have shown cause damage to our DNA and to our cells. Our cells' inability to neutralize free radicals increases with age, stress, poor nutrition and lack of exercise.

According to the laws of thermodynamics, the degree of disor-der tends to increase with the passage of time. Energy is required to prevent this process. Entropy is used to measure the degree of disorder in our bodies. We are all born captive to a disintegration process. All diseases are part of the natural result of this disin-tegration process. We could exercise right, eat super foods, use health supplements or even try plastic surgery to try to enable a long and healthy life, but eventually the negative effects of aging would catch up. Science has the potential to alter this through, among other things, the discovery of the "aging" genes.

Neurons

The primary cells of our brain are neurons, which specialize in carrying messages through an electrochemical process (synaptic firing or neuron firing). Neurons carry out almost all the activities of a normal cell except for cell division. Researchers have started to map the molecular process of memory formation and have linked the ability to remember with physical changes in neurons. They have further shown that new neurons are continually being generated from stem cells found in the hippocampus of the brain.

Neurons are functional units of the nervous system that com-municate by transmitting electrical or chemical impulses between receptors that receive stimuli and effectors that respond to stim-uli. Neurons could be sensory neurons that conduct electrical impulse toward the central nervous system and motor neurons that conduct impulses away from it. Interneurons often connect sensory neurons with motor neurons and are associated with control and coordination activities in the central nervous system. The neurons of the central nervous system influence each other with the flow of electrochemical impulses through an abundance of pathways. Neuroscientists say this could explain our enormous flexibility and capacity for information processing. A neuron has multiple extensions called dendrites, which receive incoming information that travels along the neuron to its axon, which then takes the information to the synaptic cleft, where the information is transmitted to the dendrite of the next neuron.

Voltage Gate

A neuron is like a battery, which works by changes in its voltage. Neurons, like all other cells, have a cell membrane with tiny openings that act as ion-gated pumps (for example, the sodium potassium pumps and channels that are formed by protein pores). Both pumps and channels are important factors in the body's acid-base balance, kidney functions, homeostasis and the nervous system, which all need electrical signals for communication of information and thought. The pumps are fueled by energy supplied in the form of ATP molecules and the channels operate through electrochemical gradients. The neurons rely on the pumps and the channels to maintain membrane potential and osmotic balance intracellular (within) the cell and extracellular (outside) the cell.

In particular, neurons need to increase the pumping action to transform stimulus to nerve impulse or action potential, and a significant amount of our energy in the form of ATP is used to drive this pumping action. Both pumps and channels work through voltage gates to transport sodium ions out of the cell and potassium ions into the cell. An ion has either a negative, or a positive, charged atom that is missing an electron. Voltage-gated processes maintain a negative voltage within the cell by pumping in two potassium ions for every three sodium ions it pumps outside the cell. In this way, the pumps and channels function to maintain the electrical charge in the cell, which produces action potentials or nerve impulses.

Resting Potential

When a neuron is inactive, it is said to be polarized and on a break. The neuron is in a resting potential and remains this way until a stimulus arrives. *Resting* here refers to electrical rest, not to cease working, since the cell must continue to carry out other cellular activities.

Action Potential

When a stimulus arrives at the neuron, it is receive by dendrites, which through the voltage-gated process transform the stimulus or the electrochemical signal to an action potential or nerve impulse. This nerve impulse is propagated along the neuron when sodium ions inside the neuron cause more voltage-gated channels or pumps to open laterally through the axon. This voltage-gated action moves through the neuron in a wave-like manner and propagates the nerve impulse from its receipt at the dendrite through the cell body, down the axon to the synaptic cleft.

Synapse Crossing

The synapse is the link between one neuron and another but there is no physical contact. Instead, there is a gap at the synaptic cleft. Neurons communicate through electrical and chemical signals at the synapse. When a nerve impulse reaches the synaptic cleft of a neuron, the electrical signal bridges the gap junction, which allow for more rapid communications. But usually the electrical signal is unable to cross the synaptic gap and the voltage of the action potential changes, causing calcium channels to open. This triggers the release of chemical neurotransmitters into the synaptic space. The neurotransmitter then binds to protein ions of the receiving neuron receptor. This causes the positive charge of sodium ions to trigger an electrical impulse in the receiving neuron receptor, which starts the processes again. The neurotransmitter then comes off, the receptor channel is closed and the current is turned off.

This process occurs all the time as nerve impulses travel from one neuron to the next and to the brain, from which responses travel to their final destination in the body. This obviously is a simplified version of the mechanical body brain process that contributes to our sight, hearing, tasting, feeling, perception, awareness, thought, movement and speech facilitation. The workings of our mind and mental processes are not entirely clear to science, but our subjective understanding is clear or could become clear through our own efforts.

Neurotransmitters

Researchers have isolated and named over one hundred neurotransmitters, but it is not known exactly how many of these chemical messengers exist. Some of these neurotransmitters are also hormones, and when synaptic firing occur, messages and hormones are transmitted throughout the body. It is estimated that there are some eighty-six billion neurons (some say one hundred billion) with ten thousand times as many synapses that enable signals and internal communication within our brain. Just imagine how complex this all is and when it's all working properly, such communications occur without us being aware of it. In the future, connectome should provide a full picture.

Thought Speed

The speed of the action potential does not depend on the size of the stimuli. Once a threshold of the stimuli is reached for example, the five or six photons of light in the case of the photoreceptor referred to above, the action potential is triggered regardless of how strong the stimulus is. This is known as the all-or-nothing law, because the action potential either occurs or not that is, there is no weak or partial action potential. The speed of the action potential is also not dependent on the strength of the stimulus, as it is propagated along the axon by the work of the sodium-potassium pumps or ion-gated channels.

So how do we know if a stimulus is weak or strong? The answer is the frequency and the stronger the stimulus, the greater the action potential that is set up. The frequency is a code (called the frequency code) that represents the intensity of the stimulus. The speed of the action potential would be dependent on the frequency code and the rate of propagation of the action potential along the axon.

The speed of thought also depends on whether or not the neurons are covered by a myelin sheath, which insulates and protects axons of most neurons as it sends electrical signals or impulses. Myelinated neurons speed up the action potential or nerve impulse and increase the speed of impulse propagation, which in turn speeds up our thoughts. In a myelinated axon, the action potential "jumps" from one node to the next, and the impulse propagation is rapid between the nodes. The thickest myelinated axons conduct action potential at approximately 120 meters per second.

Organ Systems

The ongoing processes that work to maintain homeostasis inside our body are at work all the time and no single mechanism works by itself. All of our body systems are at work no matter what we are doing. But depending on the activity, one or more systems may be in use more than others. Our body systems are the nervous system, the endocrine system, the integumentary system, the skeletal system, the muscular system, the respiratory system, the cardiovascular system, the immune system, the digestive system, the urinary system and the reproductive system.

The nervous system is our body's communication system, as it sends, receives and process information through electrical impulses throughout our body, telling our cells, organs and systems when and how to respond to internal and external environmental changes. Our nervous system consists of the central nervous system, which comprises of our brain and our spinal cord and the peripheral nervous system, which comprises of our voluntary nervous system (somatic) and our involuntary nervous system (autonomic). The peripheral nervous system consists of all the nerves of our body and they all enter and leave the central nervous system either through the spinal nerve, in the case of the spinal cord and the cranial nerve, in the case of the brain. The central nervous system communicates primarily through neurons and processes our thoughts.

The involuntary nervous system provides two sets of nerves throughout the body. One set comprise the sympathetic nervous system (SNS) and the other is the parasympathetic nervous system (PNS). The SNS gears the body up for short-term survival by preparing it for action in response to a signal of imminent danger. The PNS slows down the body to a relaxed mode, which happens mostly on a subconscious and involuntary level. The reflex action is an involuntary action and the response that results from a nerve impulse is called a reflex arch, which involves a sensory neuron and a motor neuron. An example of a reflex is our sudden withdrawal after we receive a pin prick. Conditioned reflexes are responses modified by past experiences, such as an awareness of danger.

The endocrine system comprises glands, which produce and release chemicals called hormones, peptides, neuropeptides and neurotransmitters. These glands regulate blood chemistry, metabolism, the growth and development of our body cells and basically every other systems of our body, thereby helping to maintain homeostasis. The glands are the hypothalamus, pituitary, thyroid, adrenal, thymus, pineal, pancreas, kidney, ovaries and testes.

Much of our body's activities are regulated by our nervous system and endocrine system and this is done mainly through the hypothalamus and the pituitary glands. The hypothalamus is in the brain at the intersection of the cortex, the cerebellum and the brainstem. It plays a key role because of the information it receives from the blood vessels passing through it and from other regions of the brain. This information is passed to the pituitary gland, which directly or indirectly through its secretion regulates the activities of all other endocrine glands.

A key homeostasis control is water and the process is called osmosis regulation. A large percentage of our body consists mainly of water, which keeps various processes in our body working at their optimum. For example, a balanced water level is critical to cell activity and to maintaining the concentration of cells' contents. Another key homeostasis control by the hypothalamus is maintaining body temperature, called thermoregulation. The enzymes that control every chemical reaction in our body work best at 37 degrees centigrade and if our cells get too hot or cold, they eventually die if they are not brought back to balance through the negative feedback process described above.

The integumentary system comprises the hair, nails, sweat glands and the largest organ in our body namely the skin. Our skin is nature's way of protecting us by forming a barrier between our internal body and the external environment. Skin maintains communications between the nervous system and the endocrine system through mechanoreceptors that detect the stimuli of touch, pain, feeling, sensations and changes in body temperature, all of which are encoded and sent to the hypothalamus via nerve impulses.

Our skin also helps to maintain homeostasis through maintaining a constant body temperature via the act of sweating if the temperature is hot or shivering if it is cold. This process is mediated through messages received from the hypothalamus gland to the skin glands through negative feedback. The skin also provides a physical barrier to prevent entry of pathogens, microbes, viruses, bacteria, fungus, noxious chemicals, radiation and foreign materials. If we injure our skin, cells are released by the immune system to heal the wound. Our skin synthesizes vitamin D from sunlight, which interacts with calcium for bone growth, but it is susceptible to damage from the ultraviolet rays of the sun. The skin provides inflammatory responses to skin injury, while healing and maintaining homeostasis. Imbalances due to stress, the effects of stress hormones and related responses are reflected in skin illness.

The skeletal system comprises the structural framework of our body, consisting of 206 bones, cartilages, ligaments, tendons and other connective tissues. The bones work with the muscular system to provide support, posture, locomotion and protection. The skeletal system provides protection for the vital organs such as our eyes, brain, heart, lungs and spinal cord, which are encased within the skeletal cavities. The skeletal system serves as a storage reserve for minerals, including calcium and phosphate. The blood's level of sodium, calcium and potassium, for example, must remain at constant levels to facilitate nerve, muscle, gland and bodily functions. When the level of minerals in the blood is low, the body uses those minerals stored in the bones. This exchange between the bone and the blood is ongoing according to the changing needs of the body, so the skeletal system plays a supportive role in the nervous, muscular and circulatory systems maintaining homeostasis.

The muscular system has three types of muscle tissues. First are the cardiac muscles, which are found only in the heart and their motion is involuntary. Second are the smooth muscles, like the muscles of the stomach and intestine, which are involuntary. The involuntary muscles are controlled automatically by the nervous system and hormones and we are often not aware that they are at work. Third are the skeletal muscles, which help our body move, walk, run and which are voluntary, meaning that we decide when to move them. The body muscles maintain a stable body temperature through the voluntary muscular activities. Movements are the main function of the muscular system which is controlled by our nervous system.

The central nervous system directs muscles to contract, expand, maintain balance and coordinate posture according to the needed response on a voluntary and involuntary basis. The muscular system supports blood and oxygen circulation through the pumping, contracting, relaxing of the heart muscles and the arteries in order to carry out blood circulation and breathing. The muscular system supports the digestive system. When food is eaten and swallowed, the voluntary muscles are at work. Thereafter the involuntary muscles work to move the food through the digestive process.

Our body muscles assist in thermoregulation to maintain normal body temperature. When it is hot, our body muscles redistribute the heat to our skin, which produces sweat and so reduces the body temperature. When it is cold, our muscles shiver involuntarily and in so doing contract to produce heat. Our muscles work when our brain sends nerve impulse from the central nervous system via the motor neurons to the muscles. This causes the muscles to contract or relax, depending on the messages sent and received.

The respiratory system is responsible for respiration, which takes place through the process of inspiration (breathing in) and expiration (breathing out). When we breathe in, air enters our body through our nostrils, nasal passages and mouth, through the pharynx, down the trachea, into the lungs via the bronchial tubes and into air sacks called alveoli, which are surrounded by a dense network of capillaries. Oxygen diffuses through the walls of the alveoli, through the capillaries and into the blood cells. Carbon dioxide follows the reverse path, diffusing from the blood to the capillaries wall through the alveoli and is then exhaled from the lungs.

Another key homeostatic control is carbon dioxide, which must be removed from our body. Otherwise, it becomes harmful as it dissolves to form an acid that can start to denature enzymes and other protein and this could cause detrimental changes in the blood's potential hydrogen (pH). Not surprisingly, therefore, the main stimulus that controls our breathing is the concentration of carbon dioxide in our blood. When carbon dioxide levels increase for example, when we consistently breathe out improperly, the chemoreceptors are stimulated and send nerve impulses to the respiratory center, the medulla in our brain. The medulla then sends out a response via a nerve impulse to the diaphragm to increase the rate of breathing so that excess carbon dioxide is exhaled. This is an involuntary process and operates by the negative feedback, which can be overridden when the rate and depth of breathing are under our voluntary control. Our breathing is controlled involuntarily and so we are not normally conscious of it. However, we can voluntarily control our breathing, as in the case of deep-breathing exercises.

The cardiovascular or circulatory system comprises the heart and miles and miles of arteries, veins, capillaries and the lymph structures, all of which are the body's transport system and are responsible for continuous blood circulation throughout our body. The heart pumps the blood, containing oxygen and nutrient, through its left side and into the aorta, the biggest artery. The aorta branches into smaller arteries and capillaries to transport this blood to all the body tissues and give nutrients and oxygen to our cells. The oxygen carried to our cells is necessary for energy production.

The blood transports waste products and carbon dioxide from our cells back to our heart, which pumps it to the lungs, where it picks up oxygen in exchange. In addition to providing our cells with oxygen and the removal of carbon dioxide, almost every other organ system relies on the cardiovascular system for the transport of nutrients, hormones, enzymes, and other bio-chemicals. The cardiovascular system also monitors the blood pressure through receptors that detect how blood vessels perform and relays this information to the brain, where action is taken to raise or lower the blood pressure. Stable and normal blood pressure is necessary to maintain homeostasis.

The immune system may be defined as our capacity to recognize when foreign material has intruded our body and to mobilize our body resources to remove that foreign material effectively from our body. In effect, it is our body's defense system against infections, bacteria and viruses. The immune system has two types of defense response systems. First is the process known as phagocytosis, in which white blood cells (phagocytes) form our body's first line of defense by engulfing invading bacteria, microorganisms and foreign particles. Second is the immune response, which is the production of antibodies in response to their recognized antigens. Our body can produce millions of different antibodies from our genes. An antigen is usually a protein molecule that can cause antibody formation. All cells contain antigens in their surface membrane that act as markers enabling cells to recognize each other. Our body can distinguish its own antigens' "self" from a foreign antigen's "non-self" and would normally only make antibodies against non-self antigens.

The digestive system's activities are coordinated by the nervous system and the endocrine system. It activates when we think of food and when we eat. Even before we eat, cranial reflexes pass through our brain as we identify sights, smells and thoughts of the food. The sensory receptors cause saliva to be secreted. This can become conditioned reflexes as we only have to think of the food for saliva to be secreted in our mouth. For example, just the thought of a juicy piece of fruit or a bar of chocolate could cause saliva to be secreted. So food enters our mouth and saliva is secreted when the taste buds stimulate nerve receptors sensitive to sweet, salty, sour, and bitter tastes. Our sensory neurons carry nerve impulses from these receptors to our brain, which sends messages via our motor neurons and nerve impulses to our salivary glands to secrete saliva.

Food is chewed, swallowed and travels down the esophagus by peristalsis to the stomach. The presence of food in our mouth and swallowing trigger nervous reflexes to pass to our brain, which sends nerve impulses via the vagus nerves to our stomach. This stimulates the gastric gland to secrete gastric juices, our liver to secrete bile and our pancreas to secrete enzymes. All of this takes place before the food reaches our stomach and preparing our stomach to receive the food. In the stomach, receptors send nerve impulses to the gastric glands, stimulating the continued flow of the gastric juices that aid digestion. Anti-acid hormones help to neutralize the acid in our stomach. Also, endocrine cells in our stomach secrete the hormone gastrin, which stimulates the gastric glands to produce a diluted form of hydrochloric acid. This makes our stomach content pH ideal for the optimal performance of the enzymes. It also kills bacteria, helps to digest proteins and aids in the digestion process.

In the small intestine, reflexes that pass through our brain inhibit secretions of gastric juice and slow the digestion process. The digested food is absorbed and transferred through the wall of the intestine and into the circulatory system. Undigested and unabsorbed food is eliminated from the body as feces. Through the actions of the hormones glucagon and insulin, the pancreas maintains a constant amount of glucose in our body. The liver assists in maintaining blood glucose levels by storing the glucose as glycogen.

All our body systems require nutrients, protein, vitamins, minerals, carbohydrates, fat and energy from the digestive system for us to survive. Another key homeostatic control is sugar, which is necessary for glucose and energy production. When we are between meals and our blood sugar is low, the hormone glucagon is released from our pancreas, which stimulates the conversion of glycogen to glucose, thereby raising our blood glucose level. On the other hand, when our blood sugar level is high, our pancreas releases the hormone insulin, which causes glucose to be removed from our blood and stored in our liver as glycogen. Our hypothalamus monitors blood sugar levels through a negative feedback loop.

The excretory system removes toxic and other waste material from our body and regulates our body fluids. The kidneys remove waste from our blood, combining it with water to form urine, which travels down two tubes called the urethra to our bladder. The urinary system is also responsible for maintaining electrolytes balance, red blood cell count and the optimum pH levels in the blood. The kidneys control the body's water levels by producing concentrated or diluted urine in response to blood plasma concentration levels that vary according to temperature, exercise, salt and fluid intakes. A key homeostatic control is urea, which is produced from the digestion of amino acids and must be removed from our body, as it is toxic.

The reproductive system contributes to homeostasis through the maintenance of the species. Eggs are produced by the ovaries in a female and sperm are produced by the testes of a male, which attempt to fertilize the egg. If successful, childbirth results.

As briefly described above, a variety of mechanisms, our cells and our organ systems work together in maintaining our body's internal environment and homeostasis. External mechanisms such as lifestyle choices and environmental factors also affect our body's ability to maintain homeostasis. These could be deficiencies caused by poor nutrition, the lack of vitamins, minerals and other nutrients. Other factors affecting homeostasis are toxins from drugs, alcohol and other substance abuse, physical imbalances due to lack of sleep, lack of sunlight, genetic makeup and mind imbalances due to anger, anxiety and fear.

First, if proper nutrition or diet does not yield the necessary and essential nutrients, protein, carbohydrates, fats, vitamins and minerals, our body will function poorly and this will result in illness and disease. Second, toxins in our body, such as insecticide, pesticides, drug and alcohol will cause cell malfunctions that lead to illnesses and diseases. Third, the maintenance of our mental or physical body through adequate sleep, sunlight and exercise is essential to prevent illness and disease. Fourth, genes we inherit can sometimes be turned off or on because of the environment or external factors, which can also lead to illness and disease. However, we should note that having certain genes is often only signifying a predisposition to a particular illness. Usually it is our lifestyle choices and environment that trigger and activate the genes' predisposition. Fifth, physical or mental health is critical, as our thoughts and emotions can cause stress, which in turn can cause illness and disease. Therefore the proper functioning of our mind and body is critical, as many diseases and illnesses can affect our cells, organs and systems and lead to early death as a result of homeostatic imbalances.

Our body is an intricate network of systems of which we do not have the complete picture as science is still making new discoveries. How then can we be responsible for such a complex system? We are not consciously involved in all the processes. Our body has an inherent and amazing ability to work in harmony to fend off challenges in order to regulate and maintain homeostasis in a changing but stable internal biochemical, physical and psychological environment that is self-regulating and rules driven. The good news is that homeostasis is a natural process of our body, so even if we don't understand its complex working at any given time, if we just follow some simple rules, our body should maintain its own balance.

We need to be aware of some simple rules: First, be mindful of proper breathing, which provides oxygen and expels carbon dioxide. Second, be mindful of stimuli that yield perceptions, thoughts, feelings and emotions. Third, be mindful of good nutrition, which yields nutrients and energy. So breathe, think and eat right. The lifestyle choices necessary to support this natural process are ours to make, whether consciously or subconsciously.

Stress Response

The stress response actively involves the endocrine system, the nervous system and the cardiovascular system, all of which are part of our body's very complex and integrated network of systems and pathways. The Hypothalamic Pituitary Adrenal Axis (HPA Axis) is a complex set of negative feedback interactions among the hypothalamus, pituitary gland, and adrenal gland. The HPA Axis is an interface between the nervous system and the endocrine system. Negative feedback loops control the hormone's release and circulation.

Neuropeptides are protein messenger molecules produced and released by neurons that act as chemical signals. Scientific research in the early 1980s discovered the neuropeptide-y neuron's axon terminal in the paraventricular nucleus present in the hypothalamus. In 1987 Haas and George conducted research that showed that neuropeptide-y activity stimulated the release of corticotrophin-releasing hormone. Here is how: we perceive a threat and this perceived thought communicates with a neuropeptide-y in a process that converts the thought to a molecule. So in this case, the thought of the threat becomes a neuropeptide-y that stimulates corticotrophin-releasing hormone (CRH), which acts as a hormone at one site and a neurotransmitter at another. How the thought turns into a neuropeptide-y has not yet been discovered and little is known about CRH, but this process starts the stress response that leads to homeostasis imbalance.

So we perceive a threat or encounter stressors (thoughts, perception and how we view situations and events). Our sympathetic nervous system (SNS) is triggered (neurons are the receptors). And our brain's HPA Axis (the control center) is activated to prepare our body for fight or flight. Here is a simplification of how it works: the thought of threat connects with the neuropeptide-y molecule in the hypothalamus gland, which then initiates the secretion of corticotrophin-releasing hormone (CRH) and vaso-pressin (AVP). The CRH and AVP, which are transported in the blood, activate the pituitary gland to release adrenocorticotropin hormone (ACTH). The ACTH travels via the bloodstream to the outer layer of the adrenal glands, situated just above the kidneys and initiates the secretion of glucocorticoid hormones (cortisol also known as hydrocortisone or corticosterone). The ACTH also activates the adrenal glands to release adrenaline (also known as noradrenaline, epinephrine, or norepinephrine).

The release of these stress hormones and the activation of the SNS responses signals the effectors namely, our heart beats faster, our blood pressure rises, we breathe faster and we release energy as our body gets ready to react to the threat or stressor. We then have plenty of energy, our senses are keener, our memory is sharper and we become less sensitive to pain, all in readiness to respond to the threat or danger. However, and most importantly, at the same time the stress hormones slow down growth and bodily functions. Our immune system responses, our digestive system and most of the other systems of our body described above do not operate at their maximum levels. This causes disruptions in our body's home-ostasis. Adrenaline, when produced frequently and excessively in response to stress, can cause the adrenal gland to become exhausted.

Ordinarily, cortisol is released into our body only occasionally. It increases our appetite and our energy levels, which enables us to carry out our daily activities. However, when cortisol levels are high, the effects can be harmful. Why? Because over time there is a buildup of stress hormones, which causes an imbalance and homeostasis is not maintained. Stress symptoms appear and our immune system becomes impaired, causing us to be susceptible to health issues. The stress hormones' activities are elevated by the onset of the stress, especially the stress that threatens physical injury, as this is often outside our thought control.

So, while the SNS is an essential mechanism that activates the stress response necessary to get us out of danger and attain short-term survival, it becomes detrimental if not turned off. Needless to say, in the long term this state cannot be good for our body and the process needs to be reversed. Our body tries to return to balance by initiating the parasympathetic nervous system (PNS), providing a relaxation response that tranquilizes and calms the nervous system, the so-called "rest and renew" or "rest and digest." This is sometimes difficult and becomes increasingly more difficult with age. It is usually a slower process than the SNS, which is immediate but more difficult to turn off. The PNS is activated by the stimulation of the vagus nerve and the release of the neurotransmitter acetylcholine.

Otto Loewi discovered in 1920 that the effect of both sympathetic and parasympathetic stimulation is mediated by the release of a chemical now called acetylcholine (ACh), the first neurotransmitter to be identified. ACh is not only responsible for relaxing and calming but also for increasing memory and learning. *Vagus* is Latin for "wandering," so called because it spreads from the brain stem to almost all the organs and organ systems of our body. It connects the brain to the body through nerve fibers and neuron pathways and uses the neurotransmitter ACh to communicate. Therefore, when the vagus nerve is activated, the relaxation and renewal response is turned on. This action is responsible for calm, peaceful and relaxing messages sent throughout our body and our heart rate and blood pressure is typically reduced.

So, when the PNS is activated, our heart rate and blood pressure returns to normal, our body become calmer and the other systems of our body resume their regular activities to regain homeostasis. A question arises: how does the body naturally speed up the activation of the PNS? Medical science has developed a process called Vagus Nerve Stimulation, which was approved by the US Food and Drug Administration (FDA). It requires a pacemaker-like implant device that sends electrical signals to the vagus nerves, which in turn activates the release of neurotransmitters. This device is used to treat epilepsy and resistant depression.

However, stress results from our perception, our conscious awareness and our mind thoughts from which electrical impulses originate. But how do perception, thoughts, and awareness originate? Well, from electric impulses, of course! It is a cycle and as said before, no one has figured out which one starts the process: the thought, the electrochemical impulse or the neuropeptides that connect with the thought.

Meanwhile we must live and cope with stress. It follows from the above that a reversal of our perceptions and our thoughts and a change of habits that trigger the stress, should reverse the stress response. So a natural way to activate the PNS is to change our thoughts, perceptions and habits. It is believed also that a natural way to stimulate the vagus nerve is through the practice of deep breathing, in which the brain communicates with the heart and the brain communicates with the bronchial tubes of the lungs via the vagus nerves and vice versa. This is a voluntary process that involves taking deep breaths from the diaphragm, which triggers the release of hormones and neurotransmitters in the vagus nerves to send messages throughout our body to calm and relax the body and thereby reduce stress. Letting go of the thoughts, feelings and emotions that caused the stress and changing your thoughts will remove the stress factor that activate the sympathetic nervous system (SNS) and create homeostasis balance. By changing your thoughts, you initiate the calm and relaxation impulse, which triggers the activation of the parasympathetic nervous system and homeostasis balance.

Stress and homeostasis are therefore at odds at different ends of the body spectrum. Stress makes us susceptible to illnesses and diseases, while homeostasis keeps us in a dynamic balance and maintains good health and wellness. So remember that stress is how you perceive it, your awareness and more importantly those thoughts. Therefore, learn to read the signs and to avoid triggers of the SNS.

In summary, we perceive through our senses and through which we observe and thoughts are formed. When we perceive signs of threat, we think we are in danger. What we perceive through the senses and the resulting thought of threat are stimuli that are transduced to nerve impulses and propagated to our brain's HPA axis. The thoughts, stimuli and nerve impulses connect with the neuropeptide-y molecules and the hypothalamus then initiates the secretion of stress hormones. So we move from thoughts in the mind to a conscious awareness through observation and perception; these intangibles through an electrochemical process is converted to tangible molecules in the hypothalamus, where the mind, the brain and the body are connected and react to the cascade of hormones and neurotransmitters released, resulting in homeostasis imbalance and stress. This is why it is believed by some, that the body-mind connection takes place at the hypothalamus.

Signs of Stress

Every person's body and mind have different capabilities and capacities and therefore responses are not necessarily the same. Consequently, the responses of the body and mind to the demand and the level of stress are different for each individual, depending on how we perceive and respond to situations. In addition, the impact of stress is different between individuals due to the fact that our body systems react differently to the slowing and shutting down of these systems during stress. Most signs of stress involve our thought process such as memory problems, an inability to concentrate, forgetfulness, a pessimistic outlook, worry about the future, failure, low self-esteem, impaired judgment and constant worrying.

We may observe signs of stress that involve our feelings and emotions, such as irritability, short temper, anxiety, nervousness, being fearful, being overwhelmed, moodiness and depression.

Then there are behavioral signs of stress, such as anger, tantrums, agitation, emotional outbursts, nervous habits like biting our lips, picking and biting our nails, grinding our teeth, heavy smoking, alcohol and drug abuse, violent and antisocial behavior and overeating or not eating.

The physical signs of stress are perspiration, increase heart rate, trembling, nervous twitches, tiring easily, sleeping difficulties, diarrhea, indigestion, vomiting, headaches, pain in the neck and back, butterflies in the stomach, weight gain and weight loss. Prolong stress can lead to depression and skin disorders, such as rashes, dermatitis, eczema, acne and psoriasis. The physical signs of stress may also be signs of medical disorders, so you should consult with your physician in this regard.

Causes of Stress

Not all situations or events in our lives are stressful. Whether they are stressful or not depends on whether we perceive them in a positive or negative manner. When we view situations and events with a negative mind-set we cannot cope and we become stressed, our body and mind then need to be reset or rebalance. The following are some of life's potentially stressful events that may or may not be stressful or may be more or less stressful, depending on one's perspective. Some major stressors are accidents, being fired from a job, bullying or harassment, competition, death of a family member, demotion, disappointments, divorce, financial problems, fights with the boss, parenting, going to a new school or university, illness, being jailed, lawsuits, marriage, menopause, moving to a new place, a new job, noise, infidelity, physical injuries, poor grades, pregnancy, retirement, serious illness, traveling, time pressure and violence. In short, just the activities of living could be stressful.

Some of the daily stresses we encounter might include arranging childcare, bad weather, car trouble, fights with a partner or family member, home maintenance and repairs, housework, homework, loud children, rude and contentious people and traffic jams. The cumulative effects of these daily activities and situations could become more stressful than the major stresses.

Therefore, the effects of stress on our daily lives are almost unavoidable and it would be ideal if we could totally avoid stress. Where we can't eliminate the effects of stress completely, we must learn to cope with it, reduce it and manage it so that we can achieve a calm and relaxed state of mind and body. Good health and wellness is predicated upon our body and mind being in homeostasis in our daily lives. However, when our body is faced with many stressors at the same time and over time, maintaining homeostasis becomes difficult, leading to illness and disease.

Stress Measurement

Since chronic stress poses such a grave danger to us, what are the diagnostic tools? Various tools exist, but they have not proven effective in determining stress levels. For example, the body's pH can be tested to measure how well our body is maintaining equilibrium. The stress test biofeedback card provides information on body temperature regulation, and this is a good indicator, but temperature is not the only mechanism that contributes to homoeostasis. The Holmes and Rahe Stress scale measures stress levels by assigning numbers to individual stressors. But this does not allow for differences in individual personalities and responses to stress and stressors, so it may not give an accurate assessment.

In early 2012, the Qualcomm Tricorder X prize was announced. It is named after the fictional cordless handheld device on *Star Trek*, which combined computer technology and imaging to diagnose when waved over a human body. According to their website, the winning X prize design would "be a tool capable of capturing key health metrics and diagnosing a set of 15 diseases. Metrics for health could include such elements as blood pressure, respiratory rate, and temperature. Ultimately, this tool will collect large volumes of data from ongoing measurements of health state through a combination of wireless sensors, imaging technologies, and portable, non-invasive laboratory replacements." Maybe the eventual diagnostic tool will be able to measure stress levels accurately also.

At this time science and medicine cannot fully define or measure and find a remedy for stress, since stress is not a disease. Today seventy-six years after Selye's GAS model for determining stress, it remains a concept not fully understood and not easily measurable. Incidentally, so does homeostasis, but that is a model we have to work with. Stress continues to cause health issues for millions of people, which no doubt is why many people are turning to complimentary, natural and holistic approaches for stress relief and stress management.

Resolve the Dilemma

The dilemma is that each individual body is made up differently. While the homoeostasis model explains how our body's cells, organs and systems work (the same building blocks for each person), they are different in how they work in each individual. This is also true of stress, the mind, consciousness and perception. So everybody has working for them the same core interrelated systems and processes namely, the body organ systems, the homoeostasis model, the brain-mind-consciousness-perception processes and the stress response. However, these systems work differently in each individual. So it seems that medicine cannot help until there is an actual malfunction resulting in disease or illness.

The mind constitutes all thoughts, consciousness constitutes acute awareness. Perception is our experiences through our awareness and senses and the body maintains life through internal self-regulation, balance and homeostasis. Therefore, for our body to function properly and for us to live a healthy life, our thoughts, awareness and the process of how we perceive things must be our main focus. Making mindful lifestyle choices and taking the action necessary to ensure internal body equilibrium and by extension, our survival is critical. So our mind thoughts, conscious awareness, and perception are keys to our survival and perhaps the most distinguishing features between us and other species. Yes, even machines may one day have brains with the same neuron circuitry as our own.

The need and indeed the onus are on each of us to become aware of our individual stress levels and our energy levels and how they affect mental and physical homoeostasis. Being mindful, observing, noticing, witnessing, becoming attuned to our body and mind and recognizing when there is a need for reset are all critical to maintaining good health and wellness. For without these, we are exposed to illnesses and diseases and by the time we get medical intervention, it may be too late to reverse the processes. Indeed, with each assault of a disease on the body and medical intervention to rectify the imbalance, our body's homoeostasis processes are weakened and it then becomes more and more difficult for the body to self-regulate.

So, with these limitations I write about no stress at the speed of thought and my stress reset. As I write, I am sure that billions of dollars are being spent worldwide on research and experimentation examining various hypotheses relating to the human-body-brain-consciousness-mind and stress, so that we as individuals can more fully understand the workings of our inner and outer world and aspire to a life of wellness, harmony, comfort, and peace on this earth.

PART IV:
THE INCREDIBLE
THOUGHT PROCESS

*Our thoughts guide our wellness, so nurture
wise thoughts.*

When we set out to get relief from stress or to reset our mind and body from stress, it is sometimes very difficult to know where, when and how to begin. We may have the best of intentions, but unless we have information and knowledge, tools and techniques, we cannot devise a plan or even begin. This book provides information for stress reset in the form of MyStress Reset Kit©, which contains four elements in our fight against the harmful effects of stress: Incredible Thought Process, MyStress Reset Tools, Insight Practices, and Mindfulness Lifestyle Plan. In this part, we will consider the Incredible Thought Process. In Part V, we will explore MyStress Reset Tools, which provide a wide range of tools from which to choose. In Part VI, you will learn about some Insight Practices like Posture (Asana), Hand position (Mudra), Deep Breathing (Pranayama), Sun Salutations (Surya Namaskara), Relaxation (Shavasana) Yogic Sleep (Yoga Nidra),

Concentration (Anapanasati), Insight Meditation (Vipassana) and Loving-Kindness and compassion (Metta). Finally, in Part VII, you will consider how to develop a Mindfulness Lifestyle Plan to suit your individual needs and it will conclude with some salient reminders about stress reset.

Thoughts to the Rescue

It's all in the thought and it really is our thoughts that guide our every conscious and our subconscious act. In May 2012 a startling and wonderful image of a smiling stroke patient in the United States appeared online. She had been paralyzed for fifteen years and she was using only her thoughts to direct a robotic arm to pick up a bottle of coffee and bring it to her lips. Research into this technology has been going on for some time and while the brain now sends signals out by a wire to the robot, maybe in the future we will see an implanted version that communicates wirelessly. Just imagine this feat is accomplished by our incredible power of thought and how wonderful it is that science and technology would be able to provide a better life for stroke and paralysis patients. But why become a patient living a debilitating lifestyle when you could avoid having a stroke by harnessing the power of your thoughts to live a lifestyle with minimum stress and maintain mind and body balance.

Thought Particles and Waves

Thoughts arise out of electrochemical action potential or nerve impulse. We often hear the expression "thought wave" and think of a soothing, relaxing and intangible state. However, if a thought is referred to as a particle, we may think of a physical form that could harm. Our thoughts transform energy to action and our energy transforms thought, which turns energy into action. As we have seen above, our thoughts create stress responses and activate relaxation responses. Therefore, our thoughts have physical and mental manifestations. So observe and be mindful of the thought particles that are intense, high energy with greater frequency and which are harmful and can result in stress. Observe and be mindful of the thought waves that are not intense, that are low energy with lower frequency and that result in relaxation and no stress.

Creative Mind

The mind is creative and our thoughts can be trained. Our thoughts create our reality, because everything we perceive in the outer world comes from within our thoughts. Our thoughts influence our conscious, our subconscious, our decisions and the minds of other people. So observe and be mindful of your thoughts. Do not engage or entertain the thought particles and focus your awareness away from them. Instead focus on and let into your mind only thought waves that brings positive results, relieve stress, and enhance your well-being.

In the Moment

Most of us go through life accepting things as we see them and adjust to situations as they arise with or without frustration, depending on how we perceive the situation. We must get a reliable fix on the idea that awareness of the present moment as reality exists only in the present moment. Our past is a thought, a memory we cannot physically change, though we could change our thoughts about it. We try to predict our future. We dream, we plan and we hope but it exists only in our thoughts and it is a thought potential. Our present is the moment we perceive, the moment we act and the moment our thought particles or thought waves are formed based on the reality of the present.

Recognize and understand thoughts and how they are perceived. Recognize and understand your perception and work with it to create your own reality, energy and action. Reduce and avoid stress at the moment that it occurs by the way you perceive stressors and your reaction to them. It is important to live in the moment, because sometimes we don't appreciate how good the moment is until it becomes a memory. So appreciate the moment and don't wait to see its value in the memory you carry of it.

Harmful Thought Particles and Beneficial Thought Waves

Have you noticed that when your thoughts are occupied with the stress, it takes your full focus, awareness and attention as you agonize over the issues? You are then operating mostly through your subconscious. You automatically carry out daily activities without mindfulness of these activities, whether it is driving, picking up your kids from school, eating or even breathing. You forget to eat properly, exercise regularly, breath properly and sleep properly. This is because your thoughts and awareness are not focused on the activity of the moment. You are focused on the stress and your thoughts are intense, high-energy thought particles. You are not mindful of the present and this is a time when a conscious effort must be made to focus on thoughtful awareness in the moment and on the task at hand. So do not engage the thought particle instead focus your awareness on the task at hand.

Every thought we have in some way emerges through transduction from stimuli to nerve impulses and links up with a group of neurons that connect with each other through synaptic firings. So the onus is on us to tap into and recognize the strength of our thoughts and train our thoughts to be thought waves, not thought particles. Through a process of analysis, we determine what is right or wrong, good or bad and liked or disliked. Through this process, our neurons communicate and through synaptic firing we create imprints that reside in our subconscious. I believe that training of our mind and consciousness can be achieved through meditation.

In due course, through research and very likely through connectome, science will understand fully how the brain and mind work. Soon the question may be how to keep our humanity, but in the meantime we must work with what we know.

The power of our thoughts is not strong in our early life. Such power is more the outcome of our ability to integrate good, bad and indifferent experiences, adversities and successes as we grow in such a way as to benefit us in our thought processes and by extension, in our daily living. In this regard, early childhood education is critical to our beliefs and thinking process. Because the conscious mind has not fully developed, the subconscious mind is impressionable. So if you tell a child that she is stupid and that she can't learn, she will think she is stupid. Her brain does not think that these are silly assertions. Just by thinking that she can't learn, a group of neurons communicate with each other and she finds that really she can't learn. It works like autosuggestion. The good news is that we can change, replace and create new groups of neurons that allow us to be smart and who we want to be.

The same holds true if you are told that you are "fat and beautiful." You then think that you are fat and beautiful and the neurons communicate with each other and you might start to overeat. The next thing you know, you are obese, suffering from bulimia and susceptible to disease. The same is true for being told that you are "fat and ugly." You might then starve and become anorexic. These thoughts fire your neurons and they are imprinted in your subconscious.

The good news is that you have the power to change your thoughts and reverse the process from thought particles to thought waves. The bad news is that the reverse process of your subconscious thought is a slower one, much like activating the parasympathetic nervous system (PNS). So there is a parallel between the sympathetic nervous system which is quick to activate and the conscious mind which is quick to change. Also there is a parallel between the

PNS which is slow to activate and the subconscious mind which is slow to change. We will look at tools and techniques that can empower you to explore the changes you need to make.

Think, Think, Think

How many times have we said, "I was only just thinking"? We are hostage and indeed a captive audience of our thoughts. The thoughts that flash through our mind in relation to our job, relationships, family, daily activities, memories, arguments, the pros and the cons totally take up our lives. This could be a good thing, but our thoughts affect how we feel not only for the better but also for the worse. Thoughts can trigger stress responses, create imbalances and hinder homeostasis. Therefore, it is crucial that we consider and recognize our thoughts as thought waves or thought particles and be able to harness the power of our thoughts effortlessly at any given time. We should have control over our thoughts, be able to analyze them and be able to identify, select and reject them.

We are constantly required to think and think! Whether it's at school, at the office or in a business, the idea is that we must think to keep in control of things and to achieve our goals and objectives. It would seem, then, that we should think less and slow down, that we should get away from the mad rush. So let's get straight to the heart of the matter: when we think less, we use less energy and we are less stressed, but when we think more, we use more energy and we are more stressed.

The question is, how do we think less in this highly complex world and achieve all that we want to achieve? How do we measure thoughts in terms of quality and not in terms of quantity? How do we become more comfortable with thinking less and producing fewer thoughts? Maybe it is simply by enjoying a state of just being without thoughts, the meditative state. Or we could go around thinking and worrying about lots of things, freak out, get anxious, get angry, get depressed, point fingers, complain, join the blame game club, start a fight and you know where this is going. On the blame game road, there is no incentive to succeed, because it is always someone else's fault that we did not succeed. This does not help us. Maybe it does in the corporate world, depending on how you view success. But does blame help us as individuals? No, because it is definitely not a solution but a problem.

Choice

The most important choice you ever have to make is what you think about. Think only about the things you need to and if you must, the things you want to. Don't give thoughts to what you don't need or want. Our proficiency in the production of thought waves as opposed to thought particles is therefore crucial to no stress and the maintenance of our health and well-being. Examine your thought particles and harness the powers within, the natural inner healing mechanism. Identify your problems, imbalances and triggers of your stress to determine the tools and techniques necessary to reset balance and to achieve a no-stress state. Remember that it could simply be your thoughts that are causing the stress and your wellness depends on the speed with which you identify these thoughts. Recognize the symptoms and identify the cause or causes. Many causes lead to the turning point or last straw and a domino effect leads to stress and imbalances.

Information

The knowledge of what causes your stress is therefore essential and powerful information to reset your imbalances. What are the thoughts that mentally and emotionally disrupt and upset you? Recognition of these indicators allows you to take steps to metabolize the stress hormones that have accumulated into harmful buildups. Once you know the real or root cause or trigger, finding the solution becomes easier. The trick is to recognize that you have a problem. Know your mind and become aware of your thoughts and how they interact with both your SNS and your PNS.

Change

Rational and irrational thoughts, emotional reasoning, all-or nothing-reasoning, seeing the negatives not the positives, thoughts of low self-esteem, seeing what we want to see and not as it really is, attempting to control and dominate others in order to feel good, complaining and blaming others, can all be identified, analyzed and controlled through the power of our thought process. We have the power to change our thoughts, to train our minds and to challenge our thoughts, even though this may be difficult and takes time, commitment and practice, but it is necessary to ensure wellness. Instead of going around feeling unhappy and blaming the world for all that ails us in life, tap into the power of your thoughts within. Become more observant and let mindful awareness be your guide. A great gift is to live in a state of awareness and to be able to live life fully with no or few regrets and recriminations.

Purification

Our incredible thought processes can be seen in their dynamic nature. Many, many thoughts flit in and out of our mind on numerous subjects every minute of every day. The secret lies in the control and purification of these thoughts working for us and not against us. Our thoughts can affect the way we perceive a threat. Also remember that our thoughts originate stress and that the activation of the SNS "gears up" our body for a fight-or-flight response. Our thoughts can eliminate stress and activate the PNS, which "gears down" our body toward relaxation.

Help in Unlikely Places

Remember, we have trillions of workers, some we have conscious control over and others we have subconscious control over. No matter what, they work mostly unsupervised and assiduously to keep you in good health and well-being. The trick is to know how and when to control, instruct and guide them to work in your best interest. Of course I am talking about our body cells and in particular our brain cells, the neurons. Science will one day be of great help in this regard, but for now you are on your own. So look, be mindful and be aware.

Awareness and Control

Self-awareness is our ability to bring thoughts to the forefront of our consciousness, to notice what we are thinking and feeling. Self-awareness of our reactions to situations, events, problems, conflicts and our mind-set is necessary for understanding our body and mind. Being aware of our body's and mind's ability and capacity to deal with such events is critical for maintaining balance and wellness. We need to be able to address stress as it occurs. Body, mind and stress reset can occur only if we are observant, mindful, opened to change and disciplined to take action when necessary.

In Control

What is self-control? The self is the mind and the body. Control is the ability to regulate. So self-control is about our mind thinking before our body acts. The challenge is to get our mind to think when it is experiencing strong thoughts and feelings like anger and to replace that feeling thought particles with peaceful thought waves. Our mind is required to control the anger and the body's immediate reaction to the anger, which would very likely to be an action we would regret. In the split second when we must replace anger with cool and collected thought waves, a trigger is needed for us to have "breathing space" before we act. I have found that this trigger is deep breathing. It is difficult at first, but if you get into the habit of breathing deeply when you are anxious or angry, it comes automatically in every situation and you won't even notice it.

You have the ability to control how you respond, to take charge of your thoughts, to change your thoughts, emotions, schedule and environment. You are able to solve problems, resolve conflicts, be peaceful and prevent stress. Sounds good, but there are those who believe that we are not in control and that how we think is predetermined. They pose the free will, determinism and fatalism arguments. The debate is ongoing and meanwhile we still have to deal with stress. Yet some prefer not to bother, because if they do, they must exercise self-control, which means making an effort to improve health and well-being.

Meditation

Meditation is a journey into our inner self from conscious thoughts to subconscious thoughts that we instinctively achieve. During meditation, the no-mind or a state of no thought is the point when we conserve energy, which remains stored. So there is no thought in the meditative state and we are not using energy. The power of our unlimited thought potential derives from our thoughts created by energy and energy created by thoughts fuels our physical world in that our body creates action and words. Our thoughts are the greatest obstacle to meditation. To achieve the meditative state we must conserve energy and thoughts by not engaging thoughts. The emphasis here is not so much on meditation in and of itself but on the outcome of the meditative state.

Introspection and Realization

Introspection, evaluation and the assessment of the self should be predicated on facts. We should aim for self-realization through the power of the thought process. Practice discrimination of thoughts through the selection and the rejection of thoughts in order to find your true self. Learn to think clearly, to regulate your mental thought process, to know what you think and to understand why you think it. Aim to understand the true nature of your life, to understand yourselves and your life's journey in this regard.

Self-reflection is an important tool. The neural circuitry of our brain enables us to live and think as individuals and in a social setting. From the time we are little until we die, we make choices and we act based on our thoughts and interactions with others. We prefer to interact with helpful and kind people and not with those who are a hindrance and vengeful. So social interaction has its advantages and disadvantages and how much or how little we interact socially depends on what works best for each individual.

Stress Management

Every person's body and mind have different capabilities and capacities. Therefore responses will not necessarily be the same. Consequently, the response to a demand will be different and the level of stress will be different. Avoiding stress is about how well our body and mind respond to the demand being placed on them. The important thing is that life should be free from disease and its debilitating effects. We should have an energized body and a relaxed mind.

Some keys to prevention and to understanding the signals received from your body and mind, are to analyze, develop your intuition, meditate and do self-inquiry. You should receive and act on positive messages. Focus on creating harmony. Moderation is the key, so you don't have to exercise to exhaustion or meditate to a trance or starve by going on stringent diets. In addition to proper breathing, practice mindfulness and good nutrition and get adequate sleep and exercise regularly.

Eliminating stress is about reversing the body and mind response to a demand it met but did not adequately deal with. Managing stress is about the inability of the body and mind to reverse the response to that unmet demand and about coping and living with the resulting stress. We attend workshops, seminars and conferences on stress management. We read and listen to inspirational speakers. However, taking action is the key to effecting changes that are necessary to reset mind, body and stress.

Medicine is concerned with telling us what is wrong with us and how to cure it and it has given us many wonderful cures. But it generally does not tell us why it went wrong and how we could have prevented it. To develop a suitable life wellness formula, you need to look within and decide what action you need to take when difficult situations arise. You need to come up with a strategy to take action when necessary. Self-awareness and self-control together are the tools that provide us with the choices we should make about how we think, act and react in different situations. So be proactive; develop a program, initiate action and continue to practice.

PART V: MY STRESS RESET TOOLS

The key to body and mind lifestyle tools is moderation.

Your goal should be to develop a lifestyle that supports stress-free living so that you will not have to deal with stress. No stress is better than stress reset! Given that stress is an unavoidable factor of daily life and may be beneficial in the short term, it seems to me that our options are to avoid stress when possible, eliminate the effects of stress as quickly as possible and manage stress when we must live with it. We need tools that can be implemented in a moment as a situation arises. Our lifestyle is the approach we take to living with the knowledge we have at our disposal to meet any contingency. Following are 105 Lifestyle Tools. All of them have merits and maybe demerits, some more than others. I have listed them in alphabetical order. So pick, choose, mix and match to arrive at your personal stress reset formula.

Lifestyle Tools

1. **Accept the Things You Can't Change**: Keep in mind the adaptation of Reinhold Niebuhr's "Serenity Prayer": "God, grant

me the serenity to accept the things I cannot change, the courage to change the things I can, and the wisdom to know the difference." Recognize instantly what you can't change in your life. Acceptance and relief will come by the very nature of recognition. For example, the death of a loved one is something we cannot change. I remember so clearly the agony and trauma on the passing of my parents and the relief that came from the words "the body is slain but the soul never dies," adapted from the *Bhagavad Gita*.

2. Accomplish Tasks: No matter how good your memory is, make a list to help you to accomplish tasks that, if left unattended, can cause you stress. Write on paper or in your computer all the tasks on your mind. This will relieve your thoughts and conserve your energy. It will also become easier to categorize, set objectives, prioritize and decide which task to start with. Crossing off the items on the list gives a sense of accomplishment and motivation to move on to the next item on the list.

Some ways to get motivated are as follows. Big tasks are not as overwhelming if broken down into small task. Start small when you undertake a big task, as we tend to procrastinate when overwhelmed by a big task. Think in terms of small steps and achieve your goal small step by step. Anticipate the joy of completion. Look forward to your success. Give yourself a reward at the completion of the task. Avoid procrastination and think of the consequences of not accomplishing the task. Look for and attempt what you love to do and the other parts of the task will get completed also. Your motivation to complete the task may be reduced if the task is boring or repetitious, so walk away and return to that task later. Identify and decide what it would take to accomplish each task. Your last resort could be to outsource the task, but this could also be your first resort.

3. Acupuncture: This is a form of traditional Chinese medicine based on a holistic approach. It explains that good health is as a result of the balance and harmony of the yin and yang extremes.

Wellness is achieved through a balance of the energy life force known as Chi, or Qi, that is said to flow on pathways or meridians through the body. An acupuncture therapist inserts needles into various parts of the body, known as acupuncture points, to access this energy flow. It is believed that when there is an imbalance, the appropriate combinations of needles at appropriate pressure points bring balance to the flow of this energy and treats the body systems.

4. Adapt to the Stressor: It is important for us to recognize and avoid contact with stressors and where this is not possible to minimize the effects of a stressful situation. Regain control of a stressful situation by changing your thoughts, expectations and attitudes toward others. It may not be possible to avoid all stressors. This could mean developing a coping strategy to adjust or to come to terms with stressful situations and stressors and to maintain your positive outlook and emotional balance. Individuals differ in their adaptation styles. Some of us are more cut and dried, while others are more flexible in removing or minimizing the role of a stressor in their life. The best course is to avoid people who constantly causes you stress and minimize your contact with them.

5. Adequate Sleep: This is sleep that ends with a spontaneous awakening and leaves us feeling refreshed and alert. Lack of sleep or insomnia, contributes to stress. Manage your time and tasks to get adequate time for sleep. Sleep is essential for good health and stress management, since without a good night's rest, your body and mind cannot operate at their optimum. Each of us has our own sleep requirement based on several factors, including genes and age. For most of us, seven to eight hours of sleep per day is sufficient. If you lose sleep one night, your body feels it the next day. If you lose sleep several nights in a row, the effects could include the impairment of your reaction time, judgment, information processing and short-term memory. You could also become moody and anxious. Avoid coffee in the evening, because it is a stimulant that can keep you up past your bedtime. If you had inadequate sleep the night before, try meditation and Yoga Nidra to reset your balance.

6. **Anger Management:** Anger is a natural emotion that comes about when we perceive an attack or threat to our well-being. The issue is mismanagement, which results in conflict and stress. Mismanaged anger can lead to domestic abuse, road rage, workplace violence and addictions, among other things. The basic strategy for managing anger is to solve problems and avoid conflict.

Techniques for dealing with the immediate anger are as follows. When you get angry, say nothing, because if you speak, it could be negative and result in conflict. Instead, focus on your breath. Breathe deeply and count to ten or one hundred, depending on how angry you are. Once you are calm and thinking clearly, express your concern in an assertive but noncontentious way. State your concern and needs clearly without controlling others or hurting them. Identify possible solutions and work on resolving the problem.

Communication is critical, so avoid heated arguments. Hold back from saying hurtful things that you will later regret. Above all, remember that you can never make everyone happy and you can never agree with everyone. You can only do your best. However, it is within your control to make yourself happy. Some people are malicious and say things to make you angry. Understand this and become indifferent to them. Treat it as beneath your dignity to acknowledge them or what they say. When you remain detached and calm and don't respond, they are likely to feel guilty, lose interest and not bother you again. You may even inspire them by your calmness. When you are angry, the best conversation you can have is with yourself, so rate the anger against the value of losing your precious peace of mind and let your inner voice allow you to take a step back. Smile to diffuse negativity caused by the anger. Insight Meditation and the Vipassana technique, addresses chronic anger.

7. Aromatherapy: This therapy uses essential oils from plants as well as ancient techniques involving candles, salts, and other products made from essential oils. The use of essential oils rubbed on the skin during massages, inhaled into the body, or diffused in the air is a holistic approach to balancing body, mind, and stress. Flowers, herbs, and spices form essences and enhance the smell through deep breathing. Put a few drops of essential oil on your hand, body, clothes and near your nose. Breathe the essence before it evaporates and feel calm and refreshed.

An aromatherapy session treats the whole you. First, you are treated to physical therapeutic massage that relieves tension and fatigue, energizes the body and soothes the skin. Second, you are treated to mental therapy with inhalation of the essential oils, which works on the brain and the nervous system, stimulating the olfactory nerve to provide soothing, calming, positive feelings and to relax the mind. The first use of aromatherapy is best done by a therapist who can also advise you on how to use aromatherapy at home. There are about 150 essential oils. A few popular ones are lavender, peppermint, eucalyptus, mint, lemon, orange, rosemary, sandalwood, cinnamon, jasmine, basil and citronella.

8. Art Therapy: This therapy uses art making and the creative process to deal with emotional issues. It is based on the theory that the creativity and self-expression involved in art help people to solve problems. Art therapy enhances physical, emotional and mental well-being. It allows your thoughts to let go of current stress, takes your mind off the stress and releases anger, anxiety and unhappiness. It is believed that being engrossed in the flow of the art to the point of being in a meditative state leaves you relaxed. It frees your thoughts, which leaves you with no stress and with a work of art. All you need is a pencil, paper, and paint. Draw a smiling face. You can't draw, just doodle with a pen or pencil on a napkin, if necessary. Rub paint on your hand and randomly rub it on paper or splash paints onto a canvas. Choose colors that suit your mood or calming colors that free your mind of thoughts.

9. Assertiveness: Assertiveness is a balance between aggression and passiveness. Will you be passive and say yes, which would result in you being taken advantage of just because you want to keep the peace and please the other person? Or will you assert what you want? When you are too passive, you send the message to others that your feelings, needs and wants are not important. This empowers them either to disregard you or to take advantage of you. If you are in a situation where you are being taken advantage of, you need to create a balance and become assertive and forthright about what you want, without being aggressive. This may mean that you have to state your position repeatedly. Eventually, the other person will realize that you are serious.

You may not always get what you want, but assertiveness builds confidence and improves your relationship with others. If you have spent years being passive, becoming assertive does not happen easily. You will need to practice. So practice saying no instead of saying yes. Saying no could be difficult, but it often prevents problems from arising. It's best to find effective methods of saying no. Stress is created when your body and mind tell you to say no but you say yes to satisfy a family member, a client or a boss. Saying no is an art that should be practiced.

10. Avoid Alcohol: When faced with difficult situations and problems, some of us seek refuge in the consumption of alcohol. While alcohol may provide short-term relief from stress, it can cause more serious health issues than stress does. Alcohol depletes your body of vitamins and other nutrients needed to keep you healthy and to relieve stress. Decisions made under the influence of alcohol can create problems and can contribute to reprehensible behavior and diseases.

Alcohol is a stressor because it stimulates the release of stress hormones, so it is best to abstain from it. However, if you don't want to abstain, keep consumption within safe limits, not only to ensure good health but also to keep within the limits stipulated by the law. Moderation is the key if you must consume alcohol.

11. Avoid Coffee: You are stressed and need a stimulant to keep your body and mind energized and alert, so a cup of coffee seems just the thing to revive you. But coffee is a stimulant because of the caffeine in it. Within five minutes of drinking coffee, your central nervous system is stimulated to produce stress hormones in your body that cause the fight-or-flight stress response. If you are already stressed, coffee makes you more stressed. Coffee also affects sleep by shortening the amount of sleep you get.

All of that said, if you are not stressed and need to stimulate analytical thinking, coffee might do the trick. One cup of coffee a day for most people may not harm them, but elevated stress hormones in the body for lengthy periods can be dangerous. So even though studies suggest that coffee contains antioxidants and may be good for you, moderation of coffee intake is the key.

12. Avoid Contentious Topics: If you feel strongly about a topic and get upset every time you discuss it, remove it from your list of conversation topics and excuse yourself every time someone brings it up. Controversial topics are generally contentious issues that everyone has different opinions and feelings about. Often they lead to heated debates and arguments that become stressful. So if you are easily stressed by debates of contentious issues such as religious, social and political beliefs, avoid such debates.

13. Avoid Comparison with Others: You are unique and different from anyone else. Your strengths and weaknesses are different so if compared with others you may or may not come out the worse. This may result in you criticizing others or singing your own praises, neither of which is desirable. You will never have enough if you always want what others have. Always wanting more is an endless cycle and you may become resentful and unhappy. Become aware of your thoughts and realize that you are comparing yourself with others. When this happens, stop yourself and focus on something else. Count your blessings and focus on your strengths and on your journey in life. Think about all the things you would like to do, to learn, or to create and about what makes you happy. You may find that you have enough and find contentment and peace in who you are and what you have.

14. Avoid Smoking: Do not smoke; it is bad for your health! People who are often stressed have a tendency to smoke and also find it difficult to quit smoking. Cigarette smoke increases carbon dioxide in the blood. Nicotine in cigarettes is a stimulant and improves the mood of the smoker for a while, but it also causes stress hormones to be produced. If you decide to stop smoking, the first problem is finding an effective way to actually stop smoking. The next problem is dealing with stress, as you will no longer be smoking to cope with stressful situations. The tools provided in this book will help you cope with stress. One of the best tools is deep breathing, because of the fact that it mimics the deep inhalation and exhalation of smoking and this gives you a sense of smoking while breathing in and breathing out, but without the harmful effects of cigarettes.

15. Avoid Relying on Others: Avoid relying on others to make you happy. Invariably, others are busy with their own lives and their own agendas. Even if you can change another person's agenda to suit your own, the time, energy, effort and resources you expend to do it is not worth the stress, anxiety and anger when others disappoint you. You would be better off utilizing your time, energies and resources in doing the things that you expect others to do for you. That way you are sure it will be done and in the way you want it done.

16. Ayurveda Natural Medicine: *Ayurveda* is Sanskrit for life science and it is perhaps the oldest form of medicine in the world, having originated in ancient India. It is founded in the belief that the individual consciousness is connected to the universal consciousness. Five elements: ether (space), air, fire, water, and earth manifest in the functioning of the five senses: taste, smell, hearing, touch and vision. If there is too much or too little of any one in the body, an imbalance occurs. The *tridosha vata* from space and air, *pitta* from fire and water and *kapha* from earth and water are believed to make up our individual constitution, called *prakuti,* which in Sanskrit means "nature." There are three qualities of nature, called *gunas.* First is *sattva,* which describes a light, clear and stable nature, denoting purity of mind and virtuous qualities that leads to awareness. Second is *rajas,* which describes an active, agitated and turbulent nature that manifests fear, worry, anger, jealousy, attachment and depression. Third is *tamasic,* which describes a heavy, dull and inert nature that manifests in actions such as violence, vindictiveness, self-destructive behavior and addiction.

Our constitution is determined at birth and each person is a combination of all three *dosha,* with a predominant *dosha* type being present at any given time. The *tridosha* govern all bodily functions, the mind and consciousness. They act as protective barriers for the body and when they are out of balance, this contributes to illness and disease. Ayurveda treatments are based on an assessment of your individual constitution and remedies attempt to redress imbalances of the *tridoshas.* Remedies include *pancha karma* (cleansing processes), Ayurveda nutrition, Yoga, herbal medication, aromatherapy, chakra therapy, color therapy, gem therapy, music therapy and home architecture. According to Ayurveda, you cannot be in good health if any one of the three *doshas* in the body, mind and soul is not in balance.

17. **Big Picture**: Look at the situation and put it in perspective. Ask yourself how important it would be to you now or in the future. If it is not that important, direct your energies elsewhere. A big-picture thinker is comfortable with ambiguity. Consider a broader outlook and varied experiences, the positive and the negative, the successes and the failures. Expand your world of thinking. Get in the habit of looking at the big picture and continually work at seeing things from a different perspective. It helps in answering the question "Why?" in problem solving.

18. Biofeedback: Biofeedback allows you to recognize your body's signals through the use of various types of equipment and is best done by a biofeedback therapist who can coach and help you to deal with stress. Biofeedback measures the body's physiological responses, such as the heart rate, muscle tension, or brain waves in real-time. Reliable equipment is necessary to this process. You are required to participate in the process, which could take many sessions.

19. Breathing Technique: Deep breathing is effective to infuse our body with oxygen and energy, to improve our mental and physical health and to provide relaxation and peace. We tend to breathe shallowly, especially when we are angry or anxious. Shallow breathing limits the amount of air and oxygen we take in.

Here is a simple deep breathing exercise. Sit up straight or lie on your back. Place your hands on your stomach and breathe in slowly and deeply through your nose, pushing your hands in with your stomach. Hold your breath to the count of three and then slowly breathe out, pushing all the air out of your body. With practice you can do deep breathing any time you feel stressed, when you simply concentrate on deeply breathing in and out. Deep breathing practices stem from Yoga Pranayama, Tai Chi, and Qi Gong. The breathing process and the respiratory system are responsible for taking oxygen to the entire body and expelling harmful toxins and carbon dioxide. When breathing is shallow, the respiratory system carries insufficient amounts of oxygen to the cells and expels insufficient carbon dioxide so detoxifying less. This leads to health issues. Simply by deep breathing, you can alleviate stress by activating the vagus nerves and the parasympathetic nervous system, thereby inducing the relaxation response.

20. Challenges: How good are we at handling stress? Our performance outcome depends in part on whether we view the stressful situation as a challenge or a threat and also depends on our coping style. Challenges are associated with positive and successful coping styles, while threats are associated with negative coping styles. It may be that the more competent we are, the more likely we are able to view any situation as a challenge rather than as a threat. So look at problems as challenges and view challenges as opportunities that can bring about growth and development.

21. Chakra: *Chakra* means "wheel" in Sanskrit and is an ancient therapy with origins in India, Tibet, China, and Japan. Chakra therapy involves the seven chakra or energy centers in the body. It is believed that when we are stressed, these energy centers are blocked. It is necessary to unblock these chakras by meditating and focusing on them so that energies can freely flow throughout the body to reduce stress. Chakra meditation is one of several methods used in Chakra therapy. The others are sound, color, gem and essential oil therapies. Chakra therapy shows you how to open your chakras and properly balance them. Sound therapy employs sound frequencies associated with each chakra to resonate and balance the chakras. The earliest sounds were created with singing bowls, which are used in sound and meditation chakra therapy. It is believed that when chakras are balanced, you feel peaceful and energized.

22. Colors: Color is a powerful tool of the advertising industry. Advertisers rely on colors to influence our minds and moods. Instead, use colors to restore and reset the balance of your mind and body to get the required mood and to relieve stress. Color therapists use a variety of techniques, advising on the colors you wear, colors in your home, your office and colors for food to get the desired results. For example, it is believed that green soothes the mind, orange lifts the spirit, white is cleansing and purifying and blue is relaxing and peaceful.

This color meditation is a simple way to relieve stress: Sit or lie in a comfortable place. Close your eyes and visualize your entire body from head to toe covered in blue light. Inhale and visualize your breath as green, and further visualize it spreading throughout your body. Exhale and visualize that the breath leaving your body is red. Now visualize your entire body covered in white light for two minutes, and then open your eyes.

23. Communication: This is a two-way process that provides opportunities for information exchange, sharing views and exploring solutions to problems. Effective communication skills help to prevent misunderstandings, mistakes, false assumptions, resentment and tension. Express yourself clearly and precisely. Listen and avoid cutting in. We all have different perspectives, so be open minded and consider other people's perspectives. Be assertive and express yourself effectively. Choose the right time to communicate. Be a responsible communicator. If you are not understood, you have not communicated effectively. Communication is the sum of our perspectives, values and motivation. Our words must align with our intentions, our values and our actions to ensure powerful communication.

24. Compartmentalization: This is where we focus on one task, problem, or event to the exclusion of all others, which are mentally compartmentalize or "boxed" as we focus on accomplishing one task. Note that these other problems are not "out of sight, out of mind." To the extent that we cannot immediately deal with a problem, compartmentalization is an effective tool to avoid stress, especially in the areas of accomplishing goals, time management, project management and problem solving.

25. Competence: Strive for competence in everything you do and use every opportunity to acquire capability and capacity. You will find that you automatically solve difficult problems because you have the capability and capacity to do so. Avoiding and coping with stress become infinitely easier.

26. Concentrate: When we are stressed, we are unable to concentrate or to focus. Every one of us has had the experience and satisfaction of working on a project with complete focus and attention as well as the frustration of not being able to concentrate and complete the project. Reset your body and mind and enhance your powers of concentration through meditation. Many forms of meditation are practiced to increase powers of concentration. Meditation is useful when we cannot focus and become restless. It brings balance to our emotions by training our mind and thoughts to focus and to concentrate.

27. Confidence: How confident are you in your ability to deal with challenges? Without self-confidence, we tend to make decisions based on fear rather than on what's best for us. Fear of failure can prevent us from being confident. So we remain in a job we hate, we move from one bad relationship to another, we never follow our dreams and we never do the things we would like to do because of our fear. Every adverse experience you overcome is a boost to your confidence and gives you strength and courage to face the next experience. This is why it is often recommended that you attempt to do the things you think you cannot do. Repeated success brings confidence. So let the fears of failure propel you into success every time. Increase your self-confidence by identifying and focusing on your talents and strengths. Really want to do something and you will enjoy doing it. Don't procrastinate, take action. Plan, prepare and rehearse for success and positive outcomes. Think confidently because it is all in the power of your thoughts. Act confidently and you will become confident.

28. Conflict Resolution: Preventing unnecessary disputes allows you to avoid stress, save time, save money and prevent damage to relationships. Disputes can be avoided by providing resolution skills to children and to adults. Acquire skills to prevent and resolve conflicts efficiently and effectively. Consider Charlie, who grew up in a household where problems were solved by quarreling and physical blows, providing nothing but more stress. Consider Joy, who grew up in a home where explanation, alternatives, verbal communication and analysis were skills used to deal with difficult situations. Joy's environment was conducive to less stress and she learned skills for coping with stress.

Conflict is an inescapable part of daily life in a complex and competitive world and negotiation can be an effective tool to resolve conflict. Among the many management styles for resolving conflicts, there are two that are most effective and best suited for stress management. First is the compromise or partial-win strategy, in which we seek solutions that partially satisfy our needs. Often this is done by splitting the difference. Second, with collaborative or win-win strategies, we seek to find solutions that fully satisfy our individual needs. This achieves an amicable settlement and gives us a sense of accomplishment, knowing that we resolved the issues without losing.

29. **Cooperate:** Help others and accept help from others. Cooperate wherever possible. Especially when you negotiate, the win-win strategy allows you to get what you want and thus reduces the incidence of stress. In business, the potential for stress is very great. The dollar is the motivating factor. Competition rules leave little room for cooperation. However cooperation can still be a useful business strategy. In family life, where the motivating factor is most often harmony, peace and happiness, cooperation is an important and achievable objective that leads to stress-free living.

30. **Dance:** Dancing is an enjoyable form of exercise that is good for the young, the old and everyone in between. When you dance, you are happier and you tend to smile and laugh more. A great amount of endorphins, the feel-good hormones, are released in your body. Dancing burns calories, increases energy, improves muscles strength and reduces stress. The benefits you receive from dancing depend on the type of dance and the consistency of practice. So put some music on. There are many entertaining dance forms to choose from, including ballroom, disco, rock and roll, folk, ballet, salsa, tango, square and belly dancing.

31. **Delegate:** Try to delegate your tasks and responsibilities or share them. If you make yourself indispensable, you have to cope with the pressures of time and demands to do more and all of this adds to stress. While delegation is a useful tool to avoid stress, if it's not done properly, it can cause even more stress. So asked yourself if the task is one you are personally responsible for or one

that can be delegated. When you delegate, give the task to a capable person and clearly explain it. To effectively delegate, make sure you give responsibility with authority and accountability.

32. Embrace Change: You have lost your job. You are recently divorced, widowed or you face some other major change in life. Stop, take stock and mother yourself. Most people resist change. But what makes them different from people who embrace change? It's all about how you perceive change. This starts at an early age. Take, for example, a child who hates going to school but her teacher makes it bearable. Then the teacher leaves at midterm and the child is sad but must accept a new teacher. The child embraces the change, realizing that at some point school ends and going to school is about the lesson learned and not only about the lesson taught. So the child had a choice to move backward, stay stagnant, or move forward. She knew she would learn nothing if she remained stagnant. If she embraced the change and learned, regardless of who was teaching, then wisdom would come.

Invariably, life does not always progress as planned, so take change in your stride. View life as an adventure, which may mean going where few others have gone before. Many new businesses start up, but few survive, because the entrepreneur must develop a business that meets market demands while making an economic return. To accomplish this, the entrepreneur must keep an open mind, view change as an opportunity, adapt and learn to meet the challenges. In short, he must embrace change. Most people become comfortable with what they do and don't expect things to change, but to improve you must do things differently, because change is a secret to success.

33. Emotional Balance: Emotional imbalance creates stress with physical manifestation. Being emotionally balanced means you are not overjoyed or upset. This is a normal state that we must constantly try to achieve. We need to be aware of our emotions, how to keep them in balance and how to bring them back into balance after a stressful situation. Emotions can range from extremely negative, such as worry, fear and anxiety, to positive, such as exhilaration, hope, eagerness and anticipation. When potentially stressful events are viewed as challenges rather than threats, we tend to exhibit better coping styles, have more positive emotional feelings and develop greater confidence. Through this we acquire self- esteem.

34. Exercise: All kinds of exercise help the body to use up excess stress hormones. An early morning walk in the park or a ten-minute walk after lunch or a thirty-minute walk in the afternoon after work can boost your immune system, relax your muscles and relieve stress. An active body promotes blood circulation and the delivery of oxygen and nutrients throughout the body, resulting in a strengthened immune system and a relaxed and stress-free body and mind. Jogging, swimming, bicycling, aerobics and the popular exercises of Tai-chi and Yoga are also beneficial.

35. Express Yourself: If you are upset, you must communicate your concerns in a polite and calm way so that your feelings are released. In this way, others can also be made aware of how you feel and can take your concerns into consideration. Express your troubles and thoughts to your family, your friends, your work colleagues and even your boss. Share your feelings, since expressing your feelings can be cathartic. Talk to a therapist. Even if there is nothing you can do to change the stress, just talking could relieve it. You may see the issue from a different perspective as you voice your thoughts. For some people, being alone is solitude, a time for quiet reflection and peace. For others, loneliness and isolation could be the cause of stress. Tell those you love or those that love you that you are having a difficult time coping with loneliness and asked for support. Talk to your pet or talk to yourself, if necessary; it may be one of the most important conversations you have.

36. Feng Shui: The ancient Chinese art of Feng Shui and the ancient Indian art of Vastu are a body of knowledge that reveals how to balance energies (*Chi* or *Qi* in Chinese and *Prana* in Sanskrit) of any given space to bring health benefits to the person inhabiting it. In short, it is about placement and is used in home and office décor to help enhance the flow of positive energy through the placement of the home, the office and the contents within. The use of color, light and crystals enhances energies of the surrounding and our physical and mental well-being. The strategic placement of objects is the key to creating natural energy flow, harmony, balance, soothing and relaxing environment.

37. **Financial Management:** Financial well-being is one goal of stress reset. Tools for securing financial well-being and acquiring financial discipline are to have a budget, save and invest to grow your assets. Identify your income, assets, and liabilities. Also prepare an annual or monthly budget, set your goals, match your expenses to your income and spend within your budget. Do this by making a list and not going over budget when shopping.

Achieving and maintaining financial management is important for reducing stress, yet most of us struggle in our attempts in this area. Track your expenses with the help of a spending diary. This does not necessarily mean that you deprive yourself but that you make wise choices. Appreciate things that money can't buy and make the most of the money you have allocated for expenses. Avoid the use of credit cards if you cannot pay the entire monthly balance, because interest rates are very high. Both working at a job and building your assets are also good ways to earn money. In short, identify and grow your income and assets while you identify and reduce your expenses and liabilities. Maintain financial health on a consistent basis so that you can reduce stress.

38. **Focus:** Focus and reflect on all the good things in your life and how lucky you are to have these blessings. Every day or every week, stop and take some time to review what you have done, what has happened in your life and what is the next step forward. Subject your behavior, experiences and thoughts to self-analysis and organization. This helps in goal planning and

accomplishment. Reflection enhances your power of awareness and analysis and your mind's activities and thoughts are kept in focus so that you can determine strategic actions. Also "converse" with yourself. Conversations with yourself and your thoughts are perhaps the most important and beneficial conversations you will have in life. In this regard, meditation or silent reflection each day is beneficial.

39. Forgiveness: When we forgive, we let go of our hurt, anger, disappointment and resentment. Forgiveness frees us from these emotions and thoughts so we are no longer captive to them and they no longer affect our sleep. Refusing to let go is insisting that the other person be the way you want him to be. Forgiving by letting go allows you to see clearly, not through your own desires. Analyze what behavior caused the hurt and prevent it from happening again. You can free yourself from the stress of disappointment, anger and resentment by forgiving and releasing negative energies. Recognize that no one is perfect and that to ere is human. Forgive and move on, but learn from the experience.

40. Gardening: Planting and reaping can bring a sense of achievement and satisfaction. Being outdoors among trees, flowers, birds, fresh air and sunlight can bring you joy and peace of mind. It can also provide necessary bodily exercise. Freshly cut grass, fruit, herbs and flowers are all refreshing and calming. Feed the birds and plant flowers. Gardens come in almost any shape and form, ranging from a garden on the grounds of your residence to house plants, to plants on a roof, on a balcony, on a patio, in an atrium, in a greenhouse or in a window box. You can plant in the ground or in pots above the ground or create a water garden in a pond with aquatic plants. Whatever your choice is, gardening is definitely therapeutic.

41. Gem or Crystal Therapy: Ancient civilizations used gems. It is believed that gemstones and crystals are therapeutic and that they radiate energy that affects the body and mind and hence can heal. This type of therapy is guided by two key concepts: the use of the highest quality gems and the use of gems cut into appropriate shapes. The therapist places crystals on different parts of the body, sometimes corresponding to the chakras, as well as around the body to construct an energy grid, surrounding you with energy. It is believed that crystals affect the electromagnetic field that surround the body, often referred to as an aura. We use crystal therapy daily when we use rock salt or table salt to season our foods. It is also believed that treating water with various crystals is therapeutic. The easiest way to do gem therapy is simply by wearing a therapeutic gem necklace, bracelet or ring. This allows energy to dissolve blockages and balance the body and mind. Pick up a gemstone and hold it tightly for a few minutes. If you feel a vibrating pulse as you squeeze, you are feeling energy pass through your body.

42. **Gratitude:** Give thanks and acknowledge the blessings you receive, both big and small. Why? Because it encourages a positive attitude and it makes you happy with who you are and what you have. Be grateful for what you have and don't worry about what you don't have. When you are grateful for the things you have, it is difficult to feel stressed about what you don't have. You are reminded to thank others and in turn receive the joy of reaching out and making someone else happy. Ingratitude alienates family members and friends and prevents you from maintaining good relationships. Many studies have shown that persons who practice daily gratitude had higher levels of alertness, enthusiasm, determination and optimism. Gratitude takes the form of a simple thank-you to someone or a formal letter of thanks. We tend to take for granted our accomplishments and all of the things we have. Keep a journal and write a list each day of the things you are grateful for. This list tends to ameliorate and put into perspective the many problems that arise.

43. **Herbal Teas:** Herbal tea, referred to by the French as *tisane,* is an infusion of spices, leaves, seeds, roots or bark in hot water. A well-brewed herbal tea provides you with plant nutrients, which

digest easily. There is a wide selection of herbal teas in health food stores and supermarkets that ease insomnia, boost the immune system, relieve anxiety and calm the nerves, such as chamomile, mint, cinnamon, peppermint, valerian, lemon balm, passion flower and rosehip. Black tea is also believed to relieve anxiety. So when you feel stressed, grab a cup of herbal tea, especially at bedtime, to relax your mind and body and to aid sleep. It is a natural way to reduces stress.

44. Hobbies: Hobbies are activities undertaken for pleasure in your spare time that can provide distraction from the stressful event. Hobbies can range from sports and games to creative activities like sewing, knitting and carpentry. Do not choose an expensive hobby (unless you could afford it) or one that might be stressful. For example, collections can be valuable to you personally and valuable to collectors. Collections are often methodically organized, cataloged and attractively and pleasingly displayed. Collectibles include stamps, coins, baseball cards, dolls and cars. Fishing and aquariums are beneficial hobbies. Watching fish play is pleasing to the eye and calming to the mind. Fishing allows you to cultivate the habit of being patient.

45. Humor and Laughter: Develop a sense of humor so you can see the funny side of everything. Make a joke, and learn to appreciate a joke. Humor distracts you from the stress. Laughter is the physiological response to humor, a powerful antidote to stress. It brings your mind and body back in balance and relaxes the whole body. It is believed that a hearty laugh relieves physical tension and stress. Laughter boosts the immune system by decreasing stress hormones and increasing immune cells and infection-fighting antibodies, thereby improving your resistance to disease. Laughter triggers the release of endorphins, the body's natural feel-good hormone. But how do you laugh when you are stressed and there is nothing funny about your stressors? Yogic laughter helps in this regard.

46. Job: Leaving your work on the job or at the office is perhaps one of the most difficult mind tasks, especially if the job is more mental than physical. The goal is to make your home free of stress relating to work. First compartmentalize and define your space and time. Set the boundaries and follow through by shutting down at the end of the workday. Turn off your computer, close the file and put it in the filing cabinet. As you leave your office, focus on how to get home and then focus on home activities. On the way home, calm your mind by listening to music or singing your favorite song. Let go of unsolved problems at work. Relieve your conscious mind by letting your subconscious mind take over the work issues. Allocate your free time to your personal and family needs and let the conscious mind become aware of these needs. When you arrive home, change out of your work clothes. Create cell phone and e-mail boundaries. Do not schedule work calls for home time unless absolutely necessary. Discourage colleagues from calling you at home to discuss work, especially in the evening as you prepare to sleep.

47. Juicing: Fresh raw fruit and vegetable juices (known as "green drink") are powerhouses of nutrients that help to improve your immune system and body functions. Vitamins are beneficial for mood, memory, mental clarity and energy. Green, leafy vegetables are a source of vitamins and minerals. Most of us do not get enough essential vitamins and minerals in our daily cooked meals. Physical health is necessary to reduce stress. Juicing provides natural vitamins and minerals, and a six-ounce glass of fresh homemade fruit and vegetable juice ensures that we get those necessary vitamins and minerals. My recipe every morning is to take one glass of fresh vegetable and fruit juice: a mixture of apple, carrot, celery, citrus fruits, sweet pepper, beet, cucumber, spinach, pineapple and watermelon. Any one or any combination is great.

48. Light Therapy: This therapy helps stimulate brain activities to reduce stress. Light therapy is done with sunlight, a light box, fluorescent light, or red light. Dim, soft lights or candlelight can create relaxing, comforting and inspirational moods. Candles come in different colors and scents. If you are doing work that involves your mental faculty, it is best to sit directly in front of a bright light.

49. **Little Pleasures:** Simple pleasures or small indulgences ease the tension of the moment. Numerous simple pleasures remind us that life is a gift and that we are alive. Such pleasures are found everywhere. Smell your favorite flowers. Enjoy clean, fresh air outdoors. Have a cup of herb tea or a small bar of dark chocolate. Enjoy the sun on your face and the wind in your hair. Take a long bath. Light incense or candles. Lie down on lavender-scented sheet. Have a quiet time of solitude. The simple pleasures are numerous and they bring joy, tranquility and peace. Identify the simple pleasures you like and keep them readily available.

50. **Love and Kindness:** Love is powerful but difficult to define. *Love* refers to many different feelings, emotions and attributes of the heart, from pleasures like loving ice cream to loving a spouse or partner. Love can be connected to the spiritual or the romantic, family, friends, pets, flowers, trees and more. Given the complexities of love and the different emotions involved, it is difficult to find a definition that clearly explains its full scope. Love is viewed as compassionate love and passionate love. It is not merely a feeling but also actions and a commitment to loving actions.

Be kind of heart and gentle with others and yourself. Love and kindness can provide a sense of security, courage and confidence and this can relieve stress. Loving family members can share your problems and offer advice, support and comfort in times of stress. Just knowing you have their support can help relieve stress. Focus on loving-kindness and compassionate thoughts to reverse harm done to the body and mind by stress.

51. **Medical Checkup:** Our body needs an annual medical checkup. Look at it as an audit, like a financial audit done at the end of the year. Call it a medical audit, if that would help you to

budget for it. Body homeostasis is critical to long-term survival. Regular medical checkups give us an indication of whether we have managed to maintain good health and wellness throughout the year.

52. Meditation: There are many meditation techniques, ancient Vedic, Buddhist, Tao, Christian other religious, nonreligious, new age and modern meditation practices. Meditation is how our thoughts and our conscious awareness are regulated during a meditation practice. The benefits of meditation are numerous, but with regard to stress, meditation brings relaxation, reflection, realization, clarity, focus, calmness and peace of mind. All of which are necessary to activate the parasympathetic nervous system. The meditation techniques that are most suited for stress are contemplation and concentration.

53. Mental Vacation: Our body automatically tenses when we get upset and our thoughts are on troubling issues. The reverse is true because when we think of good things our body feels rejuvenated and relaxed. This is because the lower center of our brain, which regulates body functions, does not distinguish between real images or imagined images.

You can reverse the effects of stress and regain balance by going on a mental vacation and on a thought-guided tour. Close your eyes and take deep breaths, while relaxing your muscles. Imagine your favorite place or scenery and imagine enjoying the smell, the sound and the taste. Imagine you are there and experiencing everything. Totally immerse yourself and you will feel good in minutes, as if you have just come back from an actual holiday.

54. Mindfulness: Focus on and observe the task at hand. If the task is physical and the mind wonders, accidents can occur and other issues can create stress. So bring your mind back to the activity at hand and continue to do this until the task is completed. This is necessary, because if the mind is focused on the activity at hand, the activity receives full attention and is satisfactorily completed. Always focus on the task or issue at hand and

"box out" other issues. Vipassana practice is a good way to develop mindfulness like this in everyday living.

55. Mind-Set: A mind-set is a set of assumptions, methods or tools we hold. It is sometimes referred to as a paradigm, which is powerful and difficult to change. In some instances, a mind-set may not be a bad thing as for example, the mind-set of a successful entrepreneur. Often our mind-set is developed as a result of our beliefs and philosophy of life. The correct mind-set to bring about change that is, positive, motivated, goal-setting mind-set is necessary for a stress-free lifestyle plan to be effective. So develop a mind-set that allows you to cope with situations and problems that could cause stress and develop the ability to focus, observe and be mindful.

56. Moderation: Moderation as opposed to excess in everything brings balance to your outer and inner life. For example, consume food and drink in moderate amounts. Exercise moderately to suit your body's needs. Spend money moderately to suit your needs and financial resources. The list goes on, because moderation is preferable to excess in almost everything we do.

57. Music: Music therapy has a tremendous effect on our body, mind and emotions. Research has shown that music with a strong beat stimulates brainwaves that resonate in sync with the beat of the music. Faster beats bring sharper concentration and more alert thinking. Slower beats promote calm and relaxation. Further, the thought-wave activity levels produced by music allow the brain to shift speed easily and have a long-lasting effect on the mind, even when the music ceases. Soothing and favorite music are powerful tools for calming the mind and heart and lifting the spirit and soul. Such music can inspire, bring understanding and transport the imagination to favorite places. Learn to sing a song, play a musical instrument and whistle a tune.

58. Nutrition: Nutrition is our body acquiring energy and nutrients needed to maintain life. A diet is the quantity and the nature of the food we eat to provide our body with the required nutrients. But we tend to become emotionally attached to foods. So, for example, when we are sad or depressed, we reach for our favorite comfort food, which is likely not a nutritious meal. So our emotions play a key role in what we eat.

Make it a habit of eating nutritious foods. Eat green, eat fresh and eat natural. Eat foods in moderate amounts, at regular intervals and with balanced nutrition to improve your health, your immune system and your ability to deal with stressful situations and events. But how do you know what to eat? The US Department of Agriculture (USDA) recently created a powerful graphical icon appropriately called MyPlate. What you put on your plate should be guided by the USDA MyPlate contents, which are vegetables and fruits on half of the plate and grains and protein on the other half of the plate, with dairy indicated by a small circle next to the plate. Make food choices that meet your needs, using the MyPlate guidelines.

When you are stressed, the temptation to eat comfort foods is great and it's easy to resort to eating a chocolate bar. We also tend not to eat or to overeat when we are under stress. The question is, how can we not turn to food for comfort and relief from stress? One of the best ways to forego junk food is not to think about it. If you redirect your conscious thought to healthy choices, when you go to the store you will automatically pick up the healthy choices you have programmed your subconscious to remember. Stress leads to a more acidic pH level, so the more alkaline the food, the more likely the body will remain in homeostasis. Remember, the ideal diet varies from individual to individual, depending on such factors as gender, age, activity, and body size.

59. **Observe:** Be in touch with your body and mind. Train your mind to observe and be aware. So many misunderstandings and disputes can be avoided if we are more observant and "pick up" on everything that can cause conflicts. Insight meditation or Vipassana is a useful tool to train your mind to automatically observe and be mindful in your daily activities.

60. Opportunity: Keep your mind open to opportunities, which can come in many disguises. If you look for opportunities in every situation, you are more likely to see them before you see threats and weaknesses. Then you have the option of choosing stress-free opportunities.

61. Patience: Being patient is an attitude that needs to be cultivated and is habit forming. For example, patience is very important when you are in a long line. Impatience can cause stress. Try to figure out why you are impatient. Pinpoint the trigger and reset to reduce the frequency of impatience. Often impatience comes when we are multitasking, on a tight schedule or stretching ourselves too thin. So consider again the to-do list you made. Do deep breathing and relaxing exercise every time you become impatient. If you can't do anything to resolve the trigger, let go and remind yourself of the bigger picture. Patience is one of the most important qualities to develop, as it helps to prevent stressful situations. Fishing is a good hobby to develop patience, because when the angler casts his fishing line, he must wait patiently for the fish to take the bait. Fishing is an art and a science and patience is a tool that must be developed for you to be a successful angler.

62. Personal Appearance and Attributes: Always dress sharply and comfortably to look good and by extension to feel good and to be confident when interacting with others. You are your own personal commercial. Look at the mirror and speak out loud about your strengths, achievements and goals. Do a one-minute résumé, which will boost your confidence and keep you in tune with what you have accomplished and your ability to do so. Reflect and be thankful for your successes. This would motivate you to achieve further successes.

Negative thoughts of ourselves can be projected to others in the form of insults and gossips. Avoid gossip and compliment others. We bring out the best of ourselves by looking for the best in others, by praising and complimenting others. So get in the habit of praising people to break the negativity cycle. Whether you are at school, work, conferences or meetings, signal your sense of confidence by sitting in front and speaking. Even if you are nervous, this allows you to build confidence and become a better public speaker.

63. Pets: In addition to or in the absence of friends and family, pets can provide excellent social support and a great way to reset your mind, body, and stress imbalance. Pets provide companionship and a feeling of warmth and they are good confidants and great listeners. Caring for pets increases our sense of responsibility. Walking is a good form of exercise for our pets and us.

64. Photo Albums and Scrapbooks: It is easy now to become a photographer. Digital technology has revolutionized the conventional camera and there are many smartphones with high-megapixel cameras, making it easier to capture beautiful pictures. But the best part is that you get to look through the lens and see different scenes and patterns, which can give you a different perspective on things around you. Home moviemaking can create and preserve beautiful memories of love, caring and stress-free living. Looking back on fond memories of happy days is a sure way to relax and reduce stress. Sitting with your photo album or scrapbook, reminiscing about family and friends and focusing on the good times causes stress to fade away. Technology has introduced digital scrapbooking and photo albums, making the memories easier to preserve for a longer time. Next time you are stressed, take pictures. It can be therapeutic.

65. Physical Appearance and Fitness: Walk briskly with confidence, even if you feel tired and depressed. The way we carry ourselves signals our well-being. If you are slouched and lethargic, this indicates a lack of confidence in what you are doing. Practice good posture and feel what it projects. Stand straight, with your shoulders squared and your head high. Make eye contact to project a positive impression. Physical fitness also greatly affects self-confidence. When we are out of shape, we feel fearful, unattractive, unsure and lacking in confidence. Let this inspire us to get the discipline to engage in physical activity.

66. **Playfulness**: Playfulness loosens you up and inspires creativity. Solving and putting together puzzles and playing board games require brain power and focus, which refreshes the mind and relieves stress. You can't pretend to be playful or fake it. Playfulness is spontaneous joyful behavior coming from within. It indicates a lightness of heart and emotional health. Playfulness occurs in the moment. Sometimes when we get caught up in stress, it is difficult to remain playful. One of the best ways to recapture playfulness is to spend time with kids. Ask them to show you a game they like. Make faces, jump, run around, play tag, or dance and in that moment you will forget your problems and stress. This is having a childlike attitude, not being childish. Childlikeness attributes like curiosity, imagination, a sense of adventure, enthusiasm, cheerfulness, an outgoing attitude and amusement, bring fun into daily life.

67. **Positive Attitude:** Cultivate a positive outlook on life and try to cope with automatic negative thoughts that surface and increase stress. Recognize that life is full of uncertainties and sometimes the best plans are subject to change due to unforeseen circumstances, so we need to cultivate a positive outlook to deal with uncertainties. Associate with a network of positive people and focus on positivity. Implement positive and inspiring thoughts. In a situation where negativity is projected, step back. It is useful to see and understand the negative aspect of a situation in order to cope and to detach yourself from the negativity. Cultivate positive thoughts when focusing on your role and goals in order to break a negativity cycle. Being positive is an attitude that must be cultivated until it becomes a habit that replaces negativity.

Your reaction to something should never be an emotional outburst. There should be a moment of silent thought and assimilation before you react. So instead of saying, "Oh no, how terrible," say nothing. At the same time, your silent, optimistic thought can be "this is an opportunity" or "I can learn or gain something from this." See the positive side in the situation. Learn to stop negative thoughts, replace them with positive thoughts and relax your mind. This can lower your stress. Look at the bright side. If you have made bad choices, reflect and learn from your mistakes.

68. Prayer: Prayer is simple and powerful. It calms the mind, gives us faith, hope, strength and courage to face adversity. Do not underestimate the power of prayer, because we may not know who God is. Prayer is an act of faith in the divinity (in whichever religion) and a communication with the universe. Prayer takes many forms, from giving thanks and worship to making request in an attempt to communicate with the divine. In moments of stress, just the repetition of a mantra, a prayer or God's name can be soothing and calming.

69. Prepared: The more information you have and can acquire about a difficult situation, the more prepared you will be and the easier it will become for you to cope. Prepare for unexpected results and unintended consequences. The more you can anticipate problems, the greater the chances are of your success. Guard against optimism, which is a good survival tool but which can create a denial of likely negative outcomes, such as "it's possible, but it can't happen." Being optimistic is natural, because you expect and see the rose-colored best and therefore don't prepare for the worst, which is likely to be the outcome. It is best to prepare for the worst and try to be realistic, so picture yourself preparing for and overcoming the worst-case scenario.

70. Preventive Maintenance: Practice preventive maintenance whenever possible, because it prevents breakdowns and failures. Carry out preventive maintenance on your house and all equipment, your car, bike, boat and yes, your body and mind. In fact, maintain anything you use that is likely to fail unexpectedly and cause you stress.

71. Proactive: Being proactive means that you foresee and anticipate difficult situations and problems and it allows you an opportunity to take evasive action and to avert danger or disaster. Being proactive also means that you plan for the future and put systems in place at home and work to make your life easier and less stressful. On a personal level, you can be proactive by nurturing your mind and body through a mindfulness lifestyle plan.

72. Problem Solving: Inherent in every situation is a problem and when our response to it causes stress, it is because of our inability to solve the problem. Don't wrestle with the problem work with it. Learn to solve problems. A problem may be fixed or treated as a challenge or an opportunity. When a problem arises, define the problem, think of alternative ways of solving the problem and select the alternative you will use. Implement the solution and then make sure that your preferred solution worked. The most difficult part is defining the problem, because if the definition is wrong, the solution will also be wrong. So it is important to know the problem and to have a clear understanding of the problem. Put the problem in perspective and answers to the why, what, how, who, when and where questions are keys to solving problems and avoiding stress. If you have a complex problem, try breaking it into smaller, manageable problems. How many different ways can you define the problem and how many different ways are available to solve the problem? If a problem arises that you cannot solve immediately, create a space in your mind and mentally "box" it until you can solve it. This prevents stress and allows you to focus on other tasks you can accomplish.

73. Progressive Muscle Relaxation: This therapy provides effective stress relief and helps if you carry the effects of stress in your body, especially your shoulders and neck. Progressive muscle relaxation may take twenty to thirty minutes to complete or just ten seconds when doing a quick tense and relaxation of a particular muscle group. Progressive muscle relaxation requires you to tighten a specific muscle group then release the muscles one at a time throughout your entire body, usually starting at your feet and working your way up to your face. During this process, notice the way your muscles feel before and after the relaxation. With practice, you will become familiar with how the tension and relaxation feel and will be able to identify stress tension when it occurs.

74. **Project Management:** You have a project, task, or goal to complete. You manage it by planning, setting objectives, organizing tasks, goals, budget, timeline and obtaining resources to complete the project or task and to achieve the goal. Project management is an effective tool for completing a project in a stress-free manner, whether it is big or small. Make a checklist of the workflow of activities and goals. Despite plans, a project can go wrong, get behind schedule or be more costly than expected, which can become very stressful. Prepare for the unexpected and prepare to solve problems as they occur. When you have many projects or many tasks within one project, compartmentalize and solve problems to reduce stress.

75. **Prioritize:** Prioritization is a necessary and important skill to ensure the balance of career, personal and family activities and relationships. It allows you to focus on matters in order of importance, to create space, to allocate time wisely and to bring order to chaos. In doing so, it reduces overall stress while you achieve your goals. Needless to say, prioritization is a key component of time management. Of course, time is not renewable, so knowing what to do and when to do it is critical. Make a master priority plan based upon your output for work, business, family, yourself, friends and others. Organize your tasks based on whether they are urgent, important, not urgent or not important. Start with an evaluation of yesterday tasks and decide today's priorities. Create your daily and weekly list. Daily prioritization complements a weekly list and you can review the weekly list every Friday afternoon.

To understand how to prioritize your tasks, you need to understand the demands on your time, money and effort as well as the input of others. Be prepared for contingencies that could delay or stall your plans and require reprioritization. Both the daily and the weekly lists should include tasks completed, not completed or reprioritized. Your master priority plan allows you never to waste time on unimportant tasks, to shape and accomplish all your goals and to limit stress.

76. Punctuality: Be punctual or even early. Being late for an appointment or meeting, even by just a few minutes, can create stress. Being late is not as inconsequential as it may seem. It signals that you lack respect for the person, occasion, or event. If this is important to you, other people's opinion of you would be a cause of stress. You then have to make excuses and apologize. The meeting has now started and you are at a disadvantage. Being punctual is a habit that extends to almost everything, including paying your bills on time, getting to work on time and arriving at school on time. A stress-free life requires that you cultivate the habit of being prompt and on time. It indicates that you are organized and can manage time effectively.

77. Quick Moves: You are sitting down and feeling tensed and stressed. Incorporate several simple, quick moves to relax your muscles. Deep breathe, get up and do three stretches. Rotate your head in a circle three times clockwise and three times counterclockwise. Shake each leg three times, jump up and down three times, and run in place for three minutes or do any other quick moves you like.

78. Read: Reading takes you anywhere you want to go. It stretches the imagination. When reading you can shut out the world, enjoy yourself, acquire knowledge and reduce stress. Focusing the mind and concentrating on written words is a distraction from stress and causes muscles to relax. Reading can become a positive form of escapism. By becoming engrossed in a book, you escape the worries and stress of the moment as your state of mind is altered by the printed words and the author's imagination. You leave your worries behind. There is an amazing and wonderful variety of material to choose from online, some of which is free. We can now carry our e-library to any part of the world, buy books, and get free books. We can read from and access this e-library anywhere, any time. It's a dream come true for avid readers.

79. Reducing Clutter: Being disorganized can be frustrating and full of tension. This is usually because you can't find things. Being disorganized also affects your ability to mentally identify and define issues and problems. So become more organized at home, at work and above all in your thoughts, which guide your actions. Reduce clutter in your life. Clean out one bit at a time. Make items easy to find by organizing them both mentally and physically.

80. Reflexology: This is a relaxation therapy and a form of complementary medicine using massage and exercise to flex the feet and hands. Reflexology therapists believe that their procedure relieves stress and that it persuades the body to correct itself biologically and achieve homeostasis balance. It is based on the principle that areas of our feet correspond to the various systems of our body. At a reflexology session, the entire foot is assessed. It is believed that applying specialized exercise and massage pressure to the foot improves the function of the various body systems.

81. Refrain from Being Influenced by Others. Don't allow other people's opinion, issues, clutter or baggage to weigh you down. Make a conscious effort to observe and become aware of the content and message in conversations. Be polite, listen and sympathize, but be free to remove what causes you stress.

82. Responsibility: Being responsible or not is how we respond to moral or legal obligations, but most of all, it is how we perceive our role in this life in relation to ourselves, our family, our employer and indeed the world. Now, this may seem like a chore or a burden. It becomes a burden for someone else to assume your responsibilities and the tendency is for everyone to think that somebody else is responsible. But responsibilities could be the opposite. They could be a pleasure and a joy. How conscious and aware we are and how we perceive and manage our life can bring a sense of fulfillment and accomplishment. Responsibilities often come with the benefits, rights, choices and opportunities of meeting challenges, doing our very best, enjoying our success, making a contribution and leaving a legacy. As J. Krishnamurti said, "You are the world and the world is you."

83. Retirement: Retirement does not mean staying at home and doing nothing. That is a recipe for disaster. Why? Because people who retire and do nothing generally become bored, depressed and morbid, worrying about death, which comes anyway, whether we worry about it or not. Revise your outlook in life by considering what to do next. Sometimes this may mean reinventing yourself. Do something you like. Make a useful and meaningful contribution as you go forward in life. Engage in fun activities, see humor in everything, laugh for no reason at all and meditate.

84. Rieki: Reiki means "life force energy." Reiki was founded by Dr. Mikao Usi, a Japanese physician. Reiki practitioners put their hands on or just above the body and move them over the body to balance energy and to facilitate positive energy flows. Reiki treatment is conducted fully clothed. You sit or lie on a couch while the healer holds her hand on or above you, moving over the organs of your body. This is said to channel universal life energy from the healer to the recipient, wherever required. There is no pressure on the body. The benefits of Reiki are said to be numerous. It relaxes the body, relieves stress and releases blocked and suppressed feelings.

85. Simplicity: One of the best ways to avoid stress is to live a life with simplicity as its goal. In a complex world with only twenty-four hours a day and even with the help of computers, internet and other technology, we can become overloaded. Lots of possessions need lots of laborious cleaning and more work. If the possessions are valuable, you need insurance and security. Stress is inevitable and we must recognize that, in the final analysis, happiness is not dependent on possessions. Our attachments to possessions and how many possessions we have acquired through the years inhibit our ability to see within ourselves and enjoy the simple pleasures of life. Simplicity can be achieved through meditation, which allows us to develop a mind that has few attachments.

86. Spa and Massage Therapies. These therapies have their origins in ancient civilizations. The term *spa* is associated with water treatment. The European spa of soaking in hot water, steaming in a vapor room and relaxing in a cooling room soothes, relaxes and rejuvenates the body and mind. Ayurveda spa therapy is designed to pamper and provide relaxation and rejuvenation for the balance of mind and body. Spa treatments are often performed at day spas, destination spas and resort spas. Treatments include natural hot springs, mineral springs, sulfur springs, hot tubs, mud baths, saunas, steam baths, aromatherapy and massages. Various massage therapies and techniques both ancient and modern are used to provide relaxation to the body muscles and to unblock energy for easy flow throughout the body.

A day at the spa can be expensive, but fortunately you can create a day spa ambience at home. Create a homemade facial from natural products like oatmeal, avocado, citrus, honey, yogurt and turmeric. Make a bubble bath with bubbles and bath salts that have relaxing properties. Add candlelight, music and aromas to your bathroom and your spa day is complete.

87. Sports and Games: A sporting activity like swimming, basketball, football, cycling, hiking, backpacking, canoeing or bowling can get your mind off work or other stressors. Children like to play games like cops and robbers, hide and seek and video games. Play Scrabble, Monopoly, card games, board games, darts and dice, to name a few. Choose the correct sport for stress reduction. If you are highly stressed, it would be best to avoid a competitive sport, as this could add to the problem. Golf can be therapeutic. Also you can pretend the ball is your problem and give it a good whacking. Try solving a crossword puzzle this occupies your mind completely and leaves no room for the stress. If you are not accustomed to physical activity, it is best to start slowly.

88. Step Back: Mentally step back from a negative situation, event or problem. Hold back an immediate response. This is easier said than done, especially when we are the subject to a verbal attack. It seems natural for us to defend ourselves and immediately get into a stressful altercation. Your first line of defense is positive thinking. An inspiring thought helps. Detach from the situation but do not withdraw completely, remain present and try to become detached while your mind finds a solution. If this does not work, you can mentally step back by practicing the physical response of actually stepping back while your mind steps back. If you are sitting, just get up, ask for an excuse and walk out. The matching of the mental step back with a physical step back creates a balance that with practice becomes automatic and allows you to deal with explosive situations with a calm and clear mind. Meditation in this regard is very helpful in training your mind to observe and be mindful.

89. Stress Balls and Worry Beads: Exercise and meditation are the main uses for the Chinese stress balls. Take the stress ball in the palm of your hand and rotate it clockwise and then counterclockwise. It is believed that stimulating the hands helps to reduce stress and promotes good health. Worry beads, called komboloi, are part of Greek culture and are unique in that they have no religious or ceremonial use. These beads are held in your hand around the forefinger and are counted by pulling downward with the thumb, which helps to relieve some of the physical tension and anxiety. Greek worry beads are simply used for relaxation and enjoyment. They generally come in odd numbers. These beads are made of any material but amber and coral are preferred because they are organic.

90. Stress Journal. Start a stress journal. All you need is pen, paper and your thoughts. Write anything that comes to your mind. This will help you identify the stressors in your life and the ways you deal with them. Writing is also a way to release stress. Each time you feel stressed, keep track of it in your journal. As you keep a daily log, you will begin to see patterns and common themes. This would help in problem solving.

91. Shiatsu: *Shiatsu* is Japanese for "finger pressure." It is the application of pressure to the body through the fingers, palms and certain techniques. It is also known as Acupressure. Shiatsu is based on traditional Japanese medicine and on the belief that illnesses are due to imbalances in the natural flow of energy, or Qi, throughout the body. Shiatsu therapists use their fingers and the palm of their hands to apply pressure in a continuous rhythmic sequence to the energy pathways, called meridians, to improve the flow of Qi. Unlike other forms of massages, no oil is applied. It is believed that Shiatsu calms the sympathetic nervous system, improves circulation, relaxes the muscles, and relieves stress.

92. Sun Salutation. *Surya Namaskara* is Sanskrit for Sun Salutation, an ancient Yoga routine. Sun Salutation is a complete Yoga technique comprising the three elements of form, energy and rhythm. It is a combination of between ten and twelve different asana, or postures, performed in specific sequence and breathing patterns, while chanting the appropriate mantra and focusing on the appropriate chakra of the body. It helps the practitioner to visualize and unblock the whole system. It stretches and tones the muscles and reduces body fat. The regular practice of Sun Salutation is believed to increase concentration levels, relieve stress and bring peace and a good night's sleep.

93. Take Control of Your Environment: Switch to a task that is not stressful while still accomplishing your goals. For example, if something on TV is stressful to watch, change the channel, watch a video or do something else. If one road has plenty of traffic, take another route. If a store is crowded and stressful, choose a time when it isn't busy. If time is a constraint, shop online. There are many alternatives to choose from when seeking to change a stressful environment.

94. **Take out Drama**: Remove drama, emotions, tears and exaggeration from your life, especially if the drama is not your concern. View situations in a drama-free way so that you are not distracted by the drama and can get to the key points immediately. Almost every time you remove drama from a situation, the issues become clearer and solutions are more evident, enabling you to remove the stress.

95. **Take Small Breaks**: Slow down and take a break from a busy and stressful situation. Often the best thing you can do is nothing. Step away from the stressor for ten minutes. Change the scenery by leaving the area. The reason for taking a break seems obvious, yet most of us think we can press on and get the work done. A short rest allows you to focus better when you return to the task at hand. A ten-minute break allows you to remove your focus from the stressful situation and put it on something else, providing rest and relaxation and increasing your capacity to respond to the stressful situation. Do some stretches or take a short walk. Do breathing exercises. Get some fresh juice or a small snack. Listen to music.

96. **Tai Chi and Qigong**: Tai Chi is an ancient Chinese, Buddhist and Taoist martial arts form. It evolved into slow, flowing and graceful postures that move smoothly one into another, transitioning into constant body motion. This is coordinated with deep breathing and directing the energy life force Chi to achieve balance and inner calm and to reduce stress. It is also called Tai Chi Chuan, which is Chinese for "supreme ultimate force." This concept is often associated with the Yin and Yang duality present in all things. Qigong, pronounced *chi kung*, is an ancient Chinese Taoist meditation involving postures slowly flowing into movement that improves and balance the body, mind and Chi. Qigong is similar to Tai Chi. The deep breathing, slow and deliberate movements and mind and body focus of Qigong, improve circulation and balance and reduce stress.

97. Time Management: Effectively manage your time to accomplish all your tasks and be stress free. When working on a big project, divide it into smaller, manageable pieces. Develop schedules, time bars and goals for each segment. This makes it manageable and less stressful. Trying to multitask is stressful and inefficient. Phone calls, texts and e-mails can be distractions, so ignore these when possible during work sessions. With poor time management, you are behind schedule and pressed for time, so it is difficult to remain calm. However, if you manage the allocated time, this can be avoided. When your time is limited, you need to compartmentalize, prioritize and focus within specific time frames to manage your time effectively.

98. Vacation: A weekend vacation is just enough time for you to relax, get peace and quiet and refresh and refocus your mind and body. Many people don't take an annual vacation. Instead, they accumulate their vacation to go on long pre-retirement leave and sometimes it is too late for this long leave to be meaningful. Even those who take annual vacations tend to take their work with them. This is unfortunate, because it keeps us in a work mind-set and therefore defeats the purpose of the vacation. A vacation allows you to relieve stress by spending time and strengthening bonds with loved ones. You enjoy free time and get restful sleep. The vacation provides an avenue for self-discovery, recovery and wellness that brings benefits long after the vacation is over.

99. Vipassana: This practice can be traced back to ancient India and was preserved by Gautama Buddha, who made it a universal practice for people of all background. *Vipassana* in the Pali language or *Vipasyana* in Sanskrit means to "see things as they really are", that is to have insight into our inner reality. It encourages us "to follow the law of nature," which Buddha called *dhamma*. Vipassana is a process of mental purification through observation of our body and mind. Seeing and becoming aware emphasizes the connection between the mind and body and allows for the transformation of our thoughts.

Vipassana is a tool used to develop, achieve and maintain mindfulness, which allows you to see things as they really are, so you do not react to anger, fear and anxiety. The Buddha said that desire and ignorance are the roots of suffering and that when these are removed, the mind becomes peaceful and happy. The benefits of practicing Vipassana are numerous, but in relation to stress, Vipassana is a key to controlling our mind and therefore our thoughts and emotions. Controlling our thoughts and emotions means that we can break addictions, craving and aversions. We can change our habits, thoughts and emotions from negative to positive, from impatience to patience, from hate to love, from agitation to calm, from anger to peace and from greed to generosity. We can think thoughts that are conducive to no-stress and mental clarity. This practice allows us to change ourselves rather than attempting the often futile task of changing others.

100. Visualization Therapy: If you cannot go on a vacation, imagine you are lying on a beach or doing a fun vacation activity of your choice. Close your eyes for ten minutes and visualize the feel of the sea, the sun and the salty air. Visualization is a form of meditation. Find a silent place, sit, close your eyes, imagine a restful scene and use all your senses to feel peace and relaxation. It is believed that through the law of attraction, visualization can lead to the realization of your dreams.

Here is how it is believed to work: Imagine and visualize your goals and dreams, leading to actually experiencing them. Your body and the universe will respond to your mind. When you visualize, you mentally rehearse solving a problem and achieving and living your goals and this leads to the real thing. Visualization allows you to rehearse mentally, to explore, to see the big picture, to receive insight and motivation and to prepare to face problems.

101. Water: Spend one hour at the beach; the lapping sound of the waves is calming. If you don't have enough time or cannot go to a beach, install a water fountain at home or a desktop fountain at the office. A water fountain improves the air quality with negative ions and acts as a humidifier. The rhythmic and rippling sound of water is soothing and reduces stress. Water makes up most of our body's total weight and is essential to a variety of functions in our body. So drink more water! We forget this basic and essential necessity, especially in times of stress.

102. Wealth: For many of us, *wealth* means lots and lots of money. For others, it means health. We so often hear the expression "health is wealth." Money is very important, but it has its place. It provides us with the necessities of life without which we would become stressed. Working at a job is a good way to make money, but there are better ways, like saving, investing and building assets. We must be aware of the distinction between attachment to wealth, desire for wealth and greed for wealth. Seeking to have money and wealth is not a problem, but it can be time consuming and stressful. The trick is to create a balance of wealth, riches, health and the pursuit of leisure and stress-free activities.

103. Yoga: This therapy is an ancient practice from India and an outstanding method of self-development and self-realization. It is one of the great ways to activate the parasympathetic nervous system, reduce stress, and create greater physical and mental harmony. Patanjali, an ancient Indian sage, propounded the Vedic concept of Yoga. In his treatise called "The Yoga Sutras," he described the eight paths of Yoga, called *Ashtangayoga,* popularly known as the "Eight Limbs of Yoga." They are *Yama*, restraints and correct social behavior; *Niyama,* inner discipline and observances; *Asana,* physical postures and practice; *Pranayama,* breath control; *Pratyahrya,* discipline of the senses; *Dharana,* concentration; *Dhyana*, meditation and *Samadhi,* self-realization and contemplation.

104. Yogic Laughter (Hasya Yoga): *Hasya* in Sanskrit means "laughter." Dr. Madan Kataria, author of the book *Laugh for No Reason* and founder and president of Laughter Clubs International is a physician who developed Laughter Yoga Therapy. Yogic laughter combines, deep controlled breathing, stretches and laughter.

You don't have to be happy to laugh and receive the same beneficial effects. It works on the basis that laughing for no reason has the same physiological effect as spontaneous laughter namely, the release of the feel-good hormone, endorphin. Deep breathing during laughter stimulates the vagus nerves and activates the parasympathetic nervous system to provide stress relief.

105. Yoga Nidra (Yogic Sleep): Swami Satyananda Saraswati developed Yoga Nidra in the mid-twentieth century from his studies of the ancient Yoga scriptures. Yoga Nidra is a method for inducing complete physical, mental and emotional relaxation. The term *Yoga Nidra* is derived from the Sanskrit words *Yoga*, meaning "union," and *nidra*, meaning "sleep." Yoga Nidra is said to be yogic sleep, meaning the body sleeps with the mind remaining awake and alert. Yoga Nidra is a deep meditation and it can be difficult to pull out of these deeper levels without the assistance of a guide. That is why a coach is recommended for beginners.

Most of these tools are fun to do and take up little time if worked into your mindful daily routine. So there is no excuse for not incorporating these necessary tools into your lifestyle.

PART VI: INSIGHT PRACTICE

Cultivate awareness in the present, don't agonize over the past or try to predict the future.

Check with your physician before starting any exercise program. The Yoga techniques provided below are intended to support the lifestyle tools above and are not for the curing of any illnesses or disease. Almost no one is too old or too out of shape to start an exercise program. Start with ten minutes a day and choose exercises that are fun to do. Also, if you find these techniques difficult to do, train first with a Yoga teacher.

These Yoga techniques provide an opportunity for you to exercise, energize, meditate, relax, harness your thoughts, and change your habits. Through changes of your thoughts and deep breathing, you can activate your parasympathetic nervous system. Really, it seems so simple: thoughts are very real because they manifest physically and mentally. They are our worst enemies when they trigger stress and our most valuable weapons when they activate relaxation. Be an officious bystander and observe your thoughts.

The following are some insight Yoga practices that I have found beneficial.

Guidelines for Practice

A certain attitude is conducive to achieving success in Yoga asana and meditation. The following are some guidelines to assist in your practice. Before practice, bathe so that you are clean and refreshed. Wear clothes that are loose and comfortable. Do not wear shoes, socks, or stockings. Sit in a place where there is fresh and clean air. Do not exercise to weariness or exhaustion. Do not rush, strain, wrestle with or aggressively do these exercises. A gentle, firm and steady effort is required. How many times have you heard the expression "go with the flow"? This works for all Yoga practices. Sit effortlessly with composure, as if time is not important. But set a specific time. Usually early in the morning is a good time. Do not expect results immediately, because success comes with patient practice

Posture or *Asana*

The following three sitting postures are in themselves therapeutic and are also used in the meditation techniques below.

Lotus Pose or *Padmasana*

Sit with your feet together, your legs fully stretched in front of you and your toes bent forward. Keep your hands at your sides with the palms touching the floor. Bend your right leg at the knee and place your right foot on the left thigh. Now bend your left leg at the knee and place your left foot on your right thigh. Your head, neck and spine are straight and erect. Your right hand is stretched out with your palms touching your right knee. Your left hand is stretched out with palms touching your left knee. Remain in this position for two minutes then come back to the original position. With every practice, try to gradually increase the time you spend in this position.

Half Lotus Pose or *Ardha Padmasana*

Sit with your feet together, your legs fully stretched in front of you and your toes bent forward. Keep your hands at your side with your palms touching the floor. Bend your right leg at your knee and place your right foot on your left thigh. Now bend your left leg at your knee and place your left foot under your right thigh. Your head, neck and spine are straight and erect. Your right hand is stretched out with your palms touching your right knee. Your left hand is stretched out with your palms touching your left knee. Remain in this position for two minutes then go back to the original position. With every practice, try to gradually increase the time you spend in this position.

Easy Pose or *Sukhasana*

Sit with your feet together, your legs fully stretched in front of you and your toes bent forward. Keep your hands at your side with your palms touching the floor. Bend one leg at the knee and place the heel under your opposite thigh. Now bend your other leg at the knee and place the heel under the opposite thigh and sit cross-legged. Your head, neck and spine are straight and erect. Your right hand is stretched out with your palms touching your right knee. Your left hand is stretched out with your palms touching your left knee. Remain in this position for two minutes then come back to the original position. With every practice, try to gradually increase the time you spend in this position.

Benefits: Among the many benefits of the above postures is relief from anxiety. It brings calm and relaxation to the mind.

Additionally, they are the recommended postures for doing meditation, as it brings composure and harmony to the body and the mind.

Hand Position or *Mudra*

The following three hand positions are in themselves therapeutic and are also used in the meditation techniques below.

A Symbol of Contemplation or *Dhyana Mudra*

Hold your hands in your lap with your left hand resting in your right hand and the tips of your thumbs touching. Your fingers should extend, pointing to the wrist of the opposite hand. The Buddha is seen holding this hand position in some pictures and statues of him.

A Handful of Flowers or *Pushpaputa Mudra*

Let your fingers rest in a relaxed position next to each other, with your thumbs against the edge of your index fingers. Then place your hands like an empty bowl on your thighs.

A Gesture of Consciousness and Knowledge or *Jnana Mudra*

Place the tip of your thumb on your index fingertip and extend all of your other fingers. Lay your right hand on your right thigh and your left hand on your left thigh with your fingers pointing up.

Benefits: The above hand positions reduce fatigue, increase vitality, clarity of mind, assertiveness and compassion.

The above Asana and Mudra are ancient practices based on Eastern philosophy that were developed to provide postures that encourage and are conducive to achieving the goals of Yoga and meditation in particular. But as we know, each of us is different mentally and physically. If these postures are difficult to achieve, don't let this deter you from developing a meditation practice. Try practicing while lying down, sitting on a chair, or even walking.

Breath Control or *Pranayama*

Pranayama is Sanskrit for "breath- control." Breathing is often done through the mouth and is often shallow. Through various subtle breathing techniques, inhaling and exhaling enhances the vital *prana*, or breath. It is difficult for most of us to control our mind. Our thoughts can adversely affect us and activate stress because we are unable to control the thoughts. The aim of *Pranayama* is to regulate our breathing to calm our mind and thoughts and to achieve relaxation. Our mind influences our breath and our breath influences our state of mind and thoughts.

Proper breathing is essential to provide our body with sufficient oxygen, a nutrient vital for the proper function of our body systems and for the elimination of carbon dioxide. Our brain requires large amounts of oxygen to function well and to prevent mental lethargy, negative thoughts and depression. Shallow breathing and breathing through the mouth limit our intake of oxygen. It is easy to breathe through your nose. Just close your mouth and automatically you will start breathing through the nose.

The yogis believed that to get the mind under control, we need to control the breath. Steady breathing brings about a steady mind, thoughts and relief from emotions, anger, frustration and anxiety. Pranayama encourages you to breathe deeply and to inhale and exhale sufficiently. So you must inhale deeply and exhale fully, slowly and evenly through the nostrils. This practice activates the parasympathetic nervous system and the vagus nerves and so relieves stress.

In Pranayama, our attention is focused on our breath and there are three key components of our breathing: First is *Puraka,* which is Sanskrit and connotes filling or completing. It describes the process of inhaling, which must be a deep and complete breath in each practice. Second is *Rechaka,* which is Sanskrit and connotes expelling or releasing. It describes the process of exhaling, which in each practice must be a complete and full release of the breath. Third is *Kumbhaka,* which is Sanskrit and connotes closing or shutting. It describes the process of retention or holding of the breath.

The following three Pranayama are effective in providing stress relief.

Alternate Nostril Breathing *(Anuloma Viloma)*

Sit in a lotus, half lotus or easy pose, whichever feels comfortable for you. Inhale through your left nostril while keeping your right nostril closed with the thumb of your right hand. Hold your breath while closing your left nostril with your third/ring finger and little finger of your right hand. Remove your thumb from your right nostril and exhale. Inhale through your right nostril while keeping your left nostril closed with the thumb of your left hand. Hold your breath while closing your right nostril with your third/ring finger and little finger of your left hand. Remove your thumb from your left nostril and exhale.

Loud Breathing or *Ujjayi*

Sit in a lotus, half lotus or easy pose, whichever feels comfortable for you. Slowly and fully inhale through both nostrils, simultaneously constricting the lower part of your tongue and the glottis. Hold your breath for about ten seconds or as long as is comfortable. Then exhale forcefully through your nostrils, creating a "whooshing" sound. Air will be forced out of your lungs. Very likely, you will find your body feeling more relaxed instantly. This is a powerful breathing and relaxation technique that creates a sense of "blowing off steam."

Bellows Breathing or *Bhastrika*

Sit in a lotus, half lotus or easy pose, whichever feels comfortable for you. Inhale and exhale quickly and rigorously for one minute, or as long as is comfortable for up to five minutes. There will be a bellowing sound while inflating and contracting your abdomen continuously, similar to the movement of a bellows. Then take a deep breath. Hold this breath for as long as it's comfortable. Then slowly and steadily exhale.

Practice Pranayama three times daily or whenever you are holding your breath or breathing shallowly because of stress, anger or frustration. Do as many repetitions of each pranayama as feels comfortable.

Sun Salutation or *Surya Namaskara*

Sun Salutation is a combination of different asana, or postures, performed in specific sequence, linking each posture with flowing and continuous movements from posture 1 through to posture 10. It stretches and tones the body muscles and reduces body fat. It also helps in deep breathing. The Ujjayi Pranayama, described above, should be used in the practice of a Sun Salutation routine. Sun Salutation is especially good if you do not have much time to devote to develop a Yoga routine. There are many different forms of Sun Salutation with slight variations in the postures. Here is a simple version, the Ashtanga Surya Namaskara (A).

This practice begins and ends with Samastithi, meaning equal standing posture and moves in a continuous flow, or *Vinyasa*, through to the end.

Start: Equal Standing Posture or *Samastithi:* Stand with your feet together, your knees straight, your head faced forward and your palms by your side. Breathe deeply.

Posture 1

Inhale and move into the *asana* called Upward Hand Pose or *Urdhva Hastasana, Ekam* (One). **Steps:** As you inhale, raise and stretch both arms out on both sides, raising them over your head and shoulders with your palms touching each other and your biceps touching your ears. Stretch your abdomen as much as possible and look up.

Posture 2

Exhale and move into the *asana* called Standing Forward Bend or *Uttanasana, Dve* (Two). **Steps:** As you exhale, bend forward and place your palms at the side of your feet, touching the floor. If this is too difficult, just touch your feet. Keep your feet straight. Touch your forehead to your knees.

Posture 3

Inhale and move into the *asana* called Half Standing Forward Bend or *Ardha Uttanasasa, Trini* (Three). **Steps:** As you inhale, move your ribs and head forward, away from your knees and look forward.

Posture 4

Exhale and move into the *asana* called Four Limb Staff Posture or *Chaturanga Dandasana, Chatvari* (Four). **Steps:** As you exhale, place your hands flat on the floor and jump or step back so that your legs and body form a straight line as you bend your elbows. Lower your body parallel to the floor, stop when your elbows are at ninety degrees and position your body so that your elbows are over your wrists.

Posture 5

Inhale and move into the *asana* called Upward Facing Posture or *Urdva Mukha Shavanasana, Panca* (Five). **Steps:** As you inhale, lower your waist, push your chest and raise your upper body. Look upward and keep your arms straight.

Posture 6

Exhale and move into the *asana* called Downward Facing Posture or *Adho Mukha Shvanasana, Shat* (Six). **Steps:** As you exhale, raise your hips and bring your head toward the floor with your eyes focus on your navel. Your body is like an inverted V. Your knees are straight and your heels are touching the floor. Remain in this posture for five deep breaths, about twenty seconds.

Posture 7

Inhale and move into the *asana* called Half Standing Forward Bend or *Ardha Uttanasana, Satpa* (Seven). **Steps:** As you inhale and keep your knees straight, jump forward straight through to your hands. Stand up with your palms at the side of your feet touching the floor and your head forward, away from your knees. Look forward.

Posture 8

Exhale and move into the *asana* called Standing Forward Bend or *Uttanasana, Ashtau* (Eight). **Steps:** As you exhale, bend forward, with your forehead touching your knees and look at your toes.

Posture 9

Inhale and move into the *asana* called Upward Hand Pose or *Urdhva Hastasana, Nava* (Nine). **Steps:** Inhale and stand straight with both hands stretched up above your head and palms clasp.

End: Equal Standing Posture or *Samastithi.* As you exhale, bring your hands to your sides with your feet together, your knee straight, your head looking forward and your palms by your sides.

This brings an end to one cycle of Sun Salutation. Do several cycles or as many as are comfortable for you. It is believed that mastering the practice of asana makes us more sensitive to our body and how it adapts and reacts. Sun Salutation is an excellent routine of a series of asana to practice that ends with a session of Yoga Nidra.

Yogic Sleep or *Yoga Nidra*

The Yogic Sleep technique should also be practiced when you feel tired and cannot concentrate during the day. It is done lying flat on your back in the Shavasana position. Yoga Nidra is a meditative practice where the body sleeps but the mind is awake and maintaining awareness on the border of sleep and wakefulness.

No experience is needed to practice Yoga Nidra, but it would be useful if your first practice session is done with a guide. With repeated practice, you should be able to get into the Yogic Sleep state at will. Yoga Nidra stimulates awareness. During Yoga nidra exactly opposite processes are used to make the brain centers active by focusing awareness on parts of the body in a sequence corresponding to various parts of the brain. Usually it takes twenty to forty minutes to complete a session.

Benefits

Yoga Nidra practice offers stress relief by providing deep relaxation, a calm state of mind, relaxation of muscles and relief from insomnia. It is believed that one hour of Yoga Nidra is equivalent to four hours of ordinary sleep. In my personal experience, it is a powerful tool for recouping lost sleep.

Relaxation or *Shavasana*

Shavasana is an asana posture and is in itself an effective technique for relief from insomnia. With practice, you will find that you either fall asleep or you enter the Yogic Sleep state.

Step 1: Internalize, relax in *Shavasana*. Lie on your back in the Shavasana posture: your eyes are lightly closed, your arms are stretch out slightly apart from your body with your palms facing upwards, your fingers are half lifted from the floor, your legs are stretch out and parted slightly and you are breathing through you nostrils quietly and naturally.

Focus your awareness on your forehead and relax. Move your awareness to your eyebrows and your eyes and relax. Move your awareness to your nostrils; settle your awareness there and relax. Move your awareness throughout your face; settle your awareness on each part and relax. Move your awareness systematically down your right shoulders, going though each part all the way to your toes in the same way: being aware, settling the awareness and relaxing. Then start at your forehead, go down your left side, doing the same as you did on the right side. Then bring your focus back to your forehead and repeat this cycle several time until your whole body feels totally relaxed.

This brings an end to the Shavasana practice, which is a prerequisite for the practice of Yoga Nidra below, but is itself beneficial, since it develops our ability to relax and to activate the parasympathetic nervous system. Attempts are also made here to slow down the sympathetic nervous system, to reset the body balance by inducing complete mental and physical relaxation. It also effectively calms the body and mind, making it more likely to fall asleep.

Yogic Sleep or *Yoga Nidra* (Continued from Step 1)

Step 2: Resolve or *Sankalpa*. Resolving is an effective way to train your thoughts and your mind processes. We are constantly being let down by people, by situations and by things, but our resolve would not fail us. Resolution creates an intention and a mental note to the subconscious mind, like autosuggestion and the creation of a seed of determination. Make a positive resolve about one of your goals, using a clear, short statement. The resolve should be to develop and strengthen the mind processes for example, "I will be free of stresses" or "I will sleep better."

Step 3: Rotation of awareness. After making the resolve, begin to visualize the part of the body mentioned by your guide. You must not move any part of your body. Quickly corresponding with the instruction, shift your awareness from one body part to the next. The whole process should be a pleasure, not a burden. You should not have any expectation or anxiety. The usual pattern is to start focusing awareness first on the right side: your thumb, fingers one by one, the palm of your hand, then your wrist, forearm, elbow, arm, shoulder, right side of your back, hip, thigh, leg, ankle, foot, big toe and other toes of the right foot. The same sequence is repeated for the left side. Then the awareness is focused on the back of your body, from the back of your head, shoulders, down your spine, thighs, heels and toes. Next be aware of the front of your body, your face, brow, eyes, nose, lips, mouth, ears, chin, neck, chest, abdomen down to your feet and toes.

Step 4: Awareness of breath. After a rotation of your consciousness of your body in sequence, focus your attention on the act of breathing to complete physical relaxation. Maintain awareness of your breath, either at your nostrils or as it passes through your throat and your belly.

Step 5: Feelings and emotions. This step brings relaxation at the level of feelings and emotions. Attempts are made to memorize the intense physical and emotional feelings; they are re-experienced, relived and then effaced. Usually this is practiced with pairs of two opposites, like hot and cold, lightness and heaviness, pain and pleasure, joy and sorrow. Relaxation at the emotional level and the building up of strong will-power are the two major outcomes of this procedure.

Step 6: Visualization. The final stage of Yoga Nidra relates to mental relaxation. Try to visualize the objects as described by your guide or any object you choose. Usually objects and symbols are chosen that have universal significance like the sun, the moon, a mountain, a river, an ocean or flowers. The practice helps to focus your mind and develop self-awareness and concentration.

Step 7: Refocus on your resolve. The resolve is intently thought of, silently repeated and even visualized. Consciously you try to direct your subconscious mind about the goal you wish to achieve. This time the subconscious mind is very receptive and therefore may accept the suggestion from the conscious mind with more intensity. It is believed that we realize our resolve in the course of time, depending upon the sincerity and regularity of the practice.

Step 8: Externalize and end the practice. Now slowly return to full awareness. Usually the instructor would guide you through the stages to come back into full awareness of the outside world.

While Yoga Nidra is very effective as a relaxation technique with many benefits for stress and insomnia, we need also to correct the triggers of stress so that we are not in a constant state of stress and relaxation modes. The next technique, Vipassana, is exceptional for correcting stress triggers in the long term.

Insight or *Vipassana*

Vipassana is taught mainly in a ten-day practice courses. However, it is a lifelong practice and you must become comfortable with it, almost for it to become second nature, if it is to impart its real value. By its very nature, we purify our thoughts and mind. But old habits die hard and impurities may return to the mind from time to time. So Vipassana has to become a way of life in order to recapture the natural law of compassion and love so its benefits can be sustained. Students must practice abstinence and undertake the five moral precepts or guidelines to correct actions, namely nonviolence, truth, non-theft, non-envy, no sexual misconduct and no use of intoxicants. Observing these precepts helps to calm the mind.

The goal is to achieve a pure mind with the highest values, leading to peace, happiness and liberation from harmful thoughts and habits. Vipassana sessions require commitment, time and discipline. It requires the ability to sit silently, the discomfort of sitting in the same position for extended periods of time and continuous practice. However, the benefits are worth the effort you put into this practice.

The Vipassana technique is simple, but the practice is very difficult and can be challenging, so a Vipassana course is recommended. Why is it difficult? Because without discipline the goal is illusive. So I could tell you that if you sit and can't focus, it is no problem, try again another time. But to get your mind to focus, you must continue to sit until your mind settles and becomes calm. This requires discipline.

The essence of Vipassana practice is the ordinary experiences of our thinking mind and our feeling body. Through our senses we hear, see, smell, taste and touch. We input our observation with total awareness or mindfulness and equanimity. The outcome is deep understanding or insight into the true nature of our experiences and purification of our thoughts.

Mindfulness means a clarity, precision and continuity of awareness. *Equanimity* means noninterference. *Insight* means wisdom gained. Purification is the whole process of gaining insights into everything, their impermanence or *anicca,* their unsatisfactory nature or *dukkha* and their lack of separate existence or transient nature or *anatta.* By our detachment and letting go of all, we gain understanding and insight.

This process is easier said than done. You must experience the observation of your mind and body in their aspects of impermanence, their unsatisfactory and transient nature. The nature of seeing that is characterized by Vipassana is that of direct perception, as distinct from knowledge derived from reading and reasoning. This practice develops a deep understanding through experience.

The process involves establishing the four foundations of mindfulness, according to the Buddhist tradition. First is the mindfulness of the body and breath, called *kaya*. Second is the mindfulness of feelings and sensations, called *vedana*. Third is the mindfulness of the mind and consciousness, called *citta*. Fourth is the mindfulness of the phenomena of nature and qualities, called *dhamma*.

Vipassana operates on the principle that sustained consciousness with equanimity of a habit breaks the habit. Equanimity is not reacting to anything, whether pleasant or otherwise, but watching everything as it is. In other words, it is an attitude of noninterference with the operation of the senses: seeing, hearing, smelling, tasting and the feeling body and the thinking mind. It is to keep balance by not to engage or not to become involved in the flow of our senses and thoughts as we watch them go by.

In our daily activities, most of us find this is very difficult to do, because reactions to our thoughts and senses are almost automatic. Have you ever noticed that if someone else has a problem, you can quickly identify the problem and find a solution; but when it's your problem, it becomes difficult? This is because you are unable to step back, to put space between you and your problem, so that you can really see it as it is. Vipassana allows you to view things objectively and dispassionately, to see them as they really are.

Vipassana is facing problems instead of ignoring or suppressing them. When we observe, face and become aware of our own negativity, anger and impure thoughts, they begin to lose their strength over us and slowly wither away.

We see anger, pleasure, happiness and more for what they are: fleeting, not created by anyone, not controlled by anyone and outside our powers to shorten or prolong. It is then we become detached; we enjoy it, but we are not attached to it. We have no desires. In so doing, we have stripped ourselves bare of our thoughts, emotions and feelings because we have seen them as they really are.

Constant practice of such insightful and mindful awareness frees us from negativity, anger and impurities. The idea is that we will have observed, watched and witnessed a gamut of experiences, thoughts, feelings, sensations and emotions without engaging them. We will have detached and let go of it all, becoming bystanders to our mind's activities: our thoughts.

The mind classifies sensation of the body as good or bad. The conscious and the subconscious mind react to it and give orders to brain neurons. Synaptic firing of the neurons sends messages to our body's organs. If we could break the cycle at this point, before orders are given to the brain, by observing the habit with equanimity, we can change it. This is the key and the challenge is to accomplish this by turning the key. However, to change the subconscious, you must experience the above by practice.

Concentration or *Anapanasati*

Part 1: Concentration

Anapanasati practice is a meditation that provides a high degree of concentration through the observance and mindfulness of the breath. Total awareness of the breath allows you to become grounded in the present moment and prevents thoughts from the past and about the future that could generate cravings or aversions and ultimately suffering. Anapanasati was expounded by the Buddha in the Great Discourse on the Foundations of Mindfulness, or the *Maha Satipatthana Sutta*. Anapanasati is a prerequisite and a part of Vipassana practice. Use a timer if necessary. Try to practice once or twice daily for one hour and at least for fifteen minutes per session.

Step 1: Sit and observe your breath, mind thoughts and body sensations.

1.1 Sit in a comfortable position with your back straight and in silence. The lotus posture or half lotus posture is preferable. If you are new to meditation, sit in the easy pose as described above. Practice finding a posture suitable to you and sit with your eyes closed.

1.2 Relax and observe the many things going on with your body, like pins and needles, numb feet, pain in the back. Observe the parade of thoughts in your mind or nothing at all. Your breathing may be fast or slow, shallow or deep. You may be breathing through your mouth or through your nostrils. Observe all thoughts and sensation. As you watch, you will notice many emotions, experiences and memories flashing by. You may focus on your thoughts and go where the thoughts carry you as you engage in the process. At the end of this session, you will have learned a lot through observation and engaging in your thought process. Keep a note of this first experience and compare it with other experiences throughout your practice. This will give you an indication of your progress.

Step 2: Observe your breath. Begin this session by sitting as in step 1.1. Close your eyes. Now breathe only through your nostrils. Inhale and exhale while observing your breath. An easy way to focus on your breath is to count one as you breathe in and two as you breathe out. Keep breathing in and out while observing your breath as it enters and leaves your nostrils. Observe as you inhale your breath, which runs from the tip of your nose, past your trachea and into your lungs.

As you focus on breathing, your mind will not always stay focused and may wander to a thought, a memory flashing by, a problem, a body sensation or pain and more, because each of our experiences are different. When this happens, observe each one with equanimity and let it fade away. Then bring your awareness back to your breath. Throughout the process, observe the experiences, the thought, the emotion, or the feeling with equanimity (without interference or engaging the thought) and bring the awareness back to your breathing time and time again. This repetitive process should at some point calm the mind and your thoughts will then focus on your body sensations. As you observe these, they too will fade away until the mind and body become calm.

Step 3: Observe and focus on your breath. Begin this session and sit, as in step 1.1. Close your eyes. Breathe as in step 2. When the mind is calm and the body comfortable observe your breath. Where is the breath entering and exiting? What sensation do you feel if any? Focus on the breath where it enters and exit your nostrils, identify the spot the air enters and exit and the sensation, hold the focus on this particular area anywhere between just above your lip and just inside your nostrils. When you identify the spot continue to focus on it trying to narrow the focus to a point. This helps to keep the focus on your breath and facilitate awareness on your breath by observing the sensations on this point with equanimity.

Step 4: Observe your breath in the present moment- Begin the session and sit as in step 1.1. Close your eyes. Breathe in and out and zero in on the point or spot where your breath enters and exits your nostrils, as in step 3. Your mind will have a lot of thoughts emerging and your body may be in pain or have other sensations. As you focus on your breath, your mind will wander and your attention will switch from your breath to your thoughts or your body, to feelings or sensations. Bring your awareness back to your breathing time and time again.

Practice watching the breath go in and out. Don't control your breathing. Watch it as it moves in and out of your nostrils. Accept the reality that your mind will wander. Bring it back again and again to your nostrils. The mind never stays in the present. It either goes to the past or tries to predict the future. Bring it back to your nostrils. Continue to refocus on your breath and eventually your mind will become calm. The goal is to achieve continuous focus and awareness in the moment on your breath, without being interrupted by your thoughts. We are all different and it may be easy or difficult for you to achieve. To some extent, this depends on how troubled or settled your mind and your experiences are at the beginning of the practice. Perfecting the habit of focus and concentration may take a week to three months or longer, depending on the variables in your practice.

This brings an end to the concentration, or *Anapanasati,* practice, which is a prerequisite for the practice of Vipassana, below, but which is in itself beneficial as it develops our power of concentration and will-power. Focusing, observing and mindfulness are the point of this part of the meditation, which is to develop deep concentration.

Part 2: Insight

Above we achieved concentration, awareness, and mindfulness of our breathing. When our thought process ceased, we acquired the tool to observe with equanimity. Now we are going to watch our thought process, our body and much more in order to gain insight.

Step 5: Observe your body from your head down. Begin the session by sitting as in step 1.1. Close your eyes and relax. Now focus your attention on the top of your head. In your mind's eye scan your entire head. If you feel sensations, do not react; observe with equanimity. Gradually and sequentially continue scanning and observing sensations from the top of your head to your feet and then begin the cycle again from the top of your head. The objective of scanning your whole body is to develop and fine-tune your skills of observation. Scanning allows you to observe your body and mind, to acquire an inner sensitivity toward all cravings and aversions and to observe them for what they are in your life.

Step 6: Observe your body from your limbs up. Begin the session by sitting as in step 1.1. Continue the process in step 5 in the reverse order that is, scan from your feet up to the top of your head. Continue to observe with equanimity. For example, if you have a sensation on your leg, just observe it. Do not interfere or engage the sensation just let it go. It may spread or it may recede and go away. Watch it as it originates and fades away. Just accept that it will inevitably pass.

Step 7: Observe your inner body from your head down, Begin the session by sitting as in step 1.1. Continue the process of scanning. Now observe the sensations inside of your body, under your skin, in your muscles and in your organs. Start from your head and move down slowly to your feet. Observe one by one each sensation with equanimity until it passes. Maintaining equanimity is critical to the success of your practice.

Step 8: Observe your inner body from your limbs up. Begin the session by sitting as in step 1.1. Continue the process of scanning and observing with equanimity as in step 7, in the reverse order from your feet up to your head.

Step 9: Observe your whole outer body. Begin the session by sitting as in step 1.1. Continue the practice of observation with equanimity. Focus on the sensation of your entire body. Watch sensations rise, recede and pass. When we observe feelings and sensations with equanimity and as they fade away, we realize that there is no suffering and we gain deep insights and understanding. We are free from suffering. We come into a deep understanding of the true nature of impermanence. We see that becoming detached and letting go changes all. The more you don't want to do something the more you do that very thing. But if we let go of all (everything that comes to our awareness) time and time again, they fade away. We gain deep insights into everything: their impermanence *(anicca)*, unsatisfactory nature *(dukka)* and their transient nature *(anatta)*. This happens when we observe with equanimity: we let go and at the point of letting go we see where we were holding on.

In that moment we gain wisdom into the impermanent, unworthy and transient nature of everything in life.

Step 10: Reflection, evaluation and outcome. Vipassana is a powerful transformation process. It trains us to become aware of the many feelings and sensations in our body and our thoughts. Watching everything, the good and the bad, with equanimity is a very difficult thing to do. It is an art and science. If you achieve it, you will be able to watch everything as you live it without reacting to it immediately and you will be able to step back when the situation demands that you do so and avoid stressful situations. You will be able to change your thoughts, habits, cravings, and aversions.

How often have you said to someone, "Don't make me angry" or "You are making me sad" or "You make me happy"? The reality is that no one can make you angry, no one can make you sad and no one can make you happy. Through Vipassana, you become aware of this reality: the wisdom and understanding that we have a choice to be angry, sad, or happy.

You may say, "Oh, but I knew all of that." Here is the problem: although we think that we know everything, we still suffer. We fail to solve problems, we fail to adequately deal with situations and we become anxious or angry at the drop of a hat. This is because true realization has to come and Vipassana practice brings this realization over time.

Vipassana practiced routinely will enable you to become conscious of your mind, thoughts, emotions, anxiety and anger as they arise and as they fade away, both while meditating and in daily life. You will come to realize that the mind and your thoughts are the source of much of the conflict you experience. The deep insights gained will give you the resilience to live a fulfilled life. You will become unaffected by the vicissitudes of life, taking it in stride and dealing with whatever curb ball is thrown your way.

Metta practice complements Vipassana because it allows us to focus on the changes we would like to make as a result of the insights gained from Vipassana practice.

Loving-kindness and Compassion Practice or *Metta Bhavana* or *Metta*
Love leaves no space for anger and hate.

Metta is a simple Buddhist technique that is simple to practice. It helps us to develop pure and positive thoughts and feelings for ourselves and for others. Remember that ATP molecules are made up of atoms, which are made up of subatomic particles. At the Quantum Mechanics level, everything is pure energy. Since we are all energy, the belief is that we are all connected and we communicate through a vibrating energy field. Metta causes a change in the energy field around us, sending ripples of energy and positive vibes that touch everybody and everything.

The result of Metta practice is inner and outer peace, love, harmony and contentment, while it facilitates thoughts of forgiveness and overcomes challenges to our forgiveness of others. It also encourages us to be kind and compassionate to all, including those who hate or dislike us. We learn to be at peace with those we disagree with and we learn to agree to disagree without ill will.

Metta practice complements Vipassana because it allows us to concentrate on the changes we would like to make within as a result of the insight gained from Vipassana. You hold to your heart and cherish phrases such as "may I be happy" and "may I be peaceful." Metta is a concentration technique, because you choose an object of concentration. Metta generates a tremendous amount of goodwill and compassion through our thoughts and intentions, which are made possible through the purification process obtained through Vipassana practice.

Step 1: Preparation. Sit in a meditative position and choose the lotus, half lotus, or easy pose. Settle yourself comfortably into the posture. Close your eyes and relax, reflect on what you would like to achieve.

Step 2: Cultivating loving-kindness and compassion. Continue and start smiling. Then focus your awareness on your heart. Breathe in and breathe out, continue to smile, be aware of your heart and focus on the center of your heart (like you focused on your breath in Vipassana). Visualize a warm glow radiating from your heart and feel the "energy" build up. Think and hold the thought of unconditional loving-kindness and compassion. If it helps, place your hand palm facing down on the area of your heart.

Step 3: Loving-kindness and compassion begins with you. Continue to breathe gently. Continue to focus on your heart and on the energies of love radiating out. Visualize the warm glow radiating from your heart and flowing throughout your body. Follow the glow radiating through your body. Say in your mind and think words of loving- kindness for you and all that you wish for yourself, like "I will find peace, love and harmony." Notice how your heart responds to this request. You will not see it, but a group of neurons is communicating through synaptic firings in your brain. Also watch the warmth of this loving intention radiate and spread throughout your body. Repeat this cycle as many times as you'd like and then return your focus to your heart.

Step 4: Loving-kindness and compassion to family members. As the last cycle ends and you return your focus to your heart in step 3 above, begin to cultivate loving-kindness and compassion as in step 2 above. Then visualize your family members and project loving-kindness and compassion to them as you did for yourself in step 3 above.

Step 5: Loving-kindness and compassion to friends and mentors. As the last cycle ends and you return your focus to your heart in step 4 above, begin to cultivate loving-kindness and compassion as in step 2 above. Then visualize your friends or mentors and project loving-kindness and compassion to them as you did for yourself in step 3 above.

Step 6: Loving-kindness and compassion to neutral persons. As the last cycle ends and you return your focus to your heart in step 5 above, begin to cultivate loving-kindness and compassion as in step 2 above. Then visualize persons you see daily but don't interact with and project loving-kindness and compassion to them as you did for yourself in step 3 above.

Step 7: Loving-kindness and compassion to difficult and hostile persons. As the last cycle ends and you return your focus to your heart in step 6 above, begin to cultivate loving-kindness and compassion as in step 2 above. Then visualize difficult persons or those who are hostile toward you and project loving-kindness and compassion to them as you did for yourself in step 3 above. Many people find the practice of Metta for hostile persons very difficult to do, but with practice you can achieve this. You may also find that your relationship with that person is improved.

Step 8: Loving-kindness and compassion to the world. As the last cycle ends and you return your focus to your heart in step 7 above, begin to cultivate loving-kindness and compassion as in step 2 above. Then visualize your town, country, the world, all living beings and project loving-kindness and compassion to them as you did for yourself in step 3 above.

Step 9: Reflections. When you complete step 8, continue to sit and reflect for a few moments on this experience. Let the loving-kindness and compassion continue to flow as you return to your daily activities.

A consistent daily practice of Deep Breathing (Pranayama), Sun Salutation (Surya Namaskara), Yogic Sleep (Yoga Nidra), Insight Meditation (Vipassana) and Loving-kindness and Compassion practice (Metta) will lead to a life without stress and with peace, tranquility, love, kindness and positivity. Does this seem too good to be true? I assure you from my personal experience that this can be achieved. When I practiced as a corporate attorney in Trinidad and Tobago some thirty years ago, the heavy workload, the anxiety and the deadlines led to elevated stress levels. At about this time my Yoga practice started and changed me as a person. It taught me to deal with anger and to cope better with the most difficult of situations.

PART VII:
A MINDFULNESS
LIFESTYLE

Life's journey begins with the first step so ensure that it's in the right direction.

Develop a Mindfulness Lifestyle Plan

When we are young, the effects of stress on homeostasis are not evident. Yet stress affects our bodily functions and the wear and tear process begins. So, if our thought process is conditioned in a particular way to arrive at stress in a given situation, we develop habits and a lifestyle that leads to early chronic stress. Ill health can happen early. By the time medical intervention is received, we are looking at a lifestyle change, which is often difficult, because we then have to break habits that have developed throughout a lifetime. Remember that stress is the demand placed on us and our inability to cope, so it can affect anyone, even children. It is therefore recommended that stress tools and techniques inform lifestyle plans and be implemented to ensure early education and development of a lifestyle that is conducive to stress-free habits.

Our lifestyle starts in infancy. How we learn, how we respond to discipline, how we solve problems, how we interact and communicate with others, as well as our thoughts, our awareness, the training of our neuron activities and the habits formed, they all begin in early childhood. Why are good parenting skills essential? Parents play a pivotal role in their children's development. Indeed, they have the power and the responsibility to nurture whole-child education and so ensure that their children become responsible adults. In addition to health and wellness, such disciplines as education and the law can critically impact childhood education, development and stress for both parents and children.

So, how do education and the law impact stress? Yes, we learn to read, write, study and take examinations to obtain certificates. Then we join the workforce. But generally we do not acquire parenting skills in this process. Of all the stresses we encounter, by far the most challenging is parenting. A recalcitrant or delinquent child is not a stressor that you as a parent can reasonably or responsibly distance yourself from. You see, it never ends for the responsible, loving and caring parents. For the irresponsible parents, the state intervenes. If those parents are uncaring, stress is not a problem for them. Indeed, such parents may be relieved when the state and/or the courts step in and relieve them of their responsibilities.

But for the loving, caring and responsible parents, getting parenting right is important for succeeding in the mission of ensuring their children become happy, productive and responsible citizens. In the lengthy process from infancy to adulthood, stress to you and to your child is inevitable. How we deal with stress depends on whether we mold responsible citizens resulting in happiness or irresponsible citizens with bad intent and resulting in lifelong stress.

The calm, cool and collected parents who can deal with any situation that arises without unnecessary panic, anger, anxiety or negative attitudes are the effective parents. They benefit from a stress-free lifestyle. Parents who are constantly angry, stressed and depressed negatively affect their children's development. You are a role model. Your inability to cope with anger, solve problems and the methods you use to resolve difficult situations, through peace or violence, are learned by your children at an early age. Developing children with a responsible mind and thoughts that peacefully solve problems or a mind that harbors bad intent is the role of the parent and the education system. Stress prevention skills should be part not only of the home curriculum but also of the school curriculum. There is no objectively correct way to raise a child, but making parenting classes compulsory ensures that everyone has access to the basic skills of parenting.

Coping with the anxiety of being a parent is a challenge for many that can lead to stress. "Family planning" is generally restricted to methods of contraception and to whether a person should become a parent or not. But family planning should actively include family nurturing and parenting. Successful parenting is an individual effort and there is no set formula. The best you can do is to ensure your child's good health, nurture his thoughts and mind, ensure the child feels loved, show care and kindness to him and develop his problem-solving skills, his self-confidence and his self-esteem.

In the beginning and in societies where living was a simple process with few options, the normal state of peace, happiness and positivity prevailed. Life was slow paced and simple, with less stress. As societies developed with more options, the faster pace and the complexity gave rise to more problems and difficult situations that resulted in stress.

Problem-solving and conflict-resolution skills are keys to developing a stress-free life. Define and solve the problems, identify and resolve the conflict as they arise and manage time adequately and wisely. For the problems you have no control over, use stress management tools to minimize the effects of stress.

A stress-free life does not require stress management tools, but it requires you to cultivate a stress-free lifestyle. This might mean using some of the tools used in stress management. They are more long lasting and effective if they become part of your day-to-day experience and are not used as quick fixes when you are "stressed out." Actually, stress will not readily arise, because these tools are part of you and are available to solve problems and resolve conflicts as they arise. Stress avoidance is a better management technique than succumbing to stress. Every time you succumb, you use one or more of the stress-relief tools, which do not necessarily solve the problem and eventually the tools become ineffective.

With age, our body cannot cope with stress and high levels of stress hormones so don't become a victim of the aging process. Consider developing a lifestyle plan that will allow you to live a stress-free life and to age with grace and dignity. Remember, it is no good if you make a plan but don't take action to implement it. Nor would it serve any useful purpose if you start a plan but don't sustain it. But how do you turn a weak, underutilized will-power or a lack of self-control into strong resolve? Remember, where attachment rules, there is no will-power, and where there is will-power, there is no attachment. Things are beautiful because of our attachment and feelings for them.

Exercising control or will-power over the mind is the key to executing a lifestyle plan successfully. Every cell in our body has a will to sustain itself, resulting in homeostasis. So too our mind also has a will, which is the ultimate purpose in life. The will to live, or self-preservation, is indeed one of our main instincts. As you age, the best motivation to develop a plan and implement it is the will to live. Laughter and positive thinking will also boost your will-power. Exercise control over your mind at every opportunity. Observe and practice mindfulness and awareness.

Since the beginning of time, people understood and were aware that the healing of our body occurs naturally by satisfying its need for balanced nutrition, pure water, fresh air, sunlight, sleep, exercise and peaceful and informed thoughts. Achieving the eight limbs of Yoga is a lifestyle plan that will assist in this regard, for it defines us as individuals in an infinite universe filled with cosmic uncertainty and in an evolving world that is fast-paced, with its fast food and and fast tracking, leaving little time to observe, savor and relax.

Be reminded of Selye's GAS and that these tools can help only in the early stages of stress. If stress becomes chronic and homoeostasis has been out of balance, early stages of illness and disease require medical intervention. So observe and be mindful of your feelings, mind and body. Listen to your body and don't hesitate to seek help. If stress is affecting the way you function, see a physician.

You may read, understand and agree with all the tools. Indeed, you may resolve to comply. Yet when it comes to implementation, you may lose the resolve. What causes us to forget all that we know for example about nutrition and how eating "comfort food" rarely gives our body the nutrients it needs? The answer is our thoughts, attachments, habits and the workings of our mind. We think that a chocolate bar tastes delicious and we become attach to it. But then it becomes a habit we can't break. The same is true of all addictions.

Before developing a lifestyle plan, consult with your physician to ensure that you are in good health and to find a way forward if you are not in good health. A wellness and lifestyle coach helps in the process of developing, implementing and evaluating a plan. A support system of family and friends helps to ensure that you complete the process. Indeed, a lifestyle plan should be a family plan.

To create a do-it-yourself lifestyle plan, consider the following.

A wellness lifestyle requires that you make good choices and conscious decisions in all areas of your life throughout each and every day. Whether you put your own needs first or last in the allocation of your time, you still need to make the right choices. Living a wellness lifestyle is important for your quality of life and your longevity. A lifestyle is a way of life and many factors influence a wellness lifestyle, including your existing way of life. Key factors are your family, job, commitments and relationships. Creating a wellness lifestyle plan is a process. The essence of developing a workable plan is to remember that you must implement it. So concentrate on the things that are within your control and the changes you want to make and are able to make.

Your personal lifestyle choices determine and inform your plan. Key inputs in figuring out and designing your plan are your strengths, weakness, needs, wants, and goals. Align your plan to your day-to-day activities. This makes it easier to incorporate in your daily life. Commit to your plan and feel good about yourself as part of the plan. Make it a family endeavor to assist in implementing and sticking to your plan, but remember you must implement it.

During the implementation of your plan, consider the outcomes and get feedback from family and friends on how you are doing. The insights gained into success or failure can pave the way to continued effort. A simple plan and knowledge of how to bring balance in your life will allow great results. However, changing your lifestyle is not a quick process and it requires practice and commitment.

Conclusion

Achieve inner peace and minimize outer chaos.

Peace of mind is something we all value and want. A few of us get it. Some of us get it fleetingly and most of us are in a state of restlessness. So how do we achieve peaceful thoughts amid chaos? We can learn to cultivate and achieve peace of mind by following a few techniques summarized from the above lifestyle tools, as follows:

Except if we see someone break the law, which we must report to the authorities, we mind our own business. We forgive the person who insults us so that we can remove ill will from our hearts. We do not look at what others have. We are not all the same and our levels of achievements are different. We reason that what we have is enough to make us happy and we focus on our own goals. We believe in ourselves and don't crave recognition and praise from others, who would then have the ability to control our peace of mind any time they withheld praise. We adapt to and become harmonious with our environment, however unfriendly. We endure what we cannot change and learn to be cheerful about it. We don't assume or take more responsibility than we are capable of carrying. We do not procrastinate or have regrets. We learn from our mistakes but don't agonize over the past. We keep our mind occupied with positive thoughts and our body with worthwhile activities. To help us achieve this, we exercise and practice meditation and Vipassana to achieve insights and attain peace of mind. We choose our thoughts and create our own wellness.

Our thoughts, beliefs, and habits can be changed with commitment and persistence. To make a change and to take action, we must act in the now, in the present. Wellness depends on our lifestyle, which in turn depends on the choices we make, which are informed by our perceptions, thoughts, and awareness. Maintaining wellness at the speed of thought is that simple. Our past is a thought, a memory we cannot physically change, though we can change our thoughts about it. Our future is our hopes, dreams and predictions of what it will be. It exists only in our thoughts; it is a thought potential. Our present is the moment we perceive and so now is the only time to act, to change our thoughts and our reality. "Right here right now!" You have the tools and techniques. You have the choice.

In the final analysis, we must think qualitative thoughts to avoid frequently activating our sympathetic nervous system (SNS). A frequently activated SNS builds up stress hormones, resulting in stress and stress-related illnesses and diseases. But you have another chance if your thoughts get the better of you and your SNS is frequently activated: breathe deeply, meditate and change your perceptions, thoughts and habits to activate your parasympathetic nervous system. This will bring calm and relaxation, which will relieve stress. So my mantra is breathe deep, eat natural, love all, sleep, laugh, pray, observe, be mindful and above all, nurture wise thoughts.

MyStress Reset Kit© has guided me to live a relatively stress-free life. Develop your own lifestyle plan from MyStress Reset Kit©. Try each one of the lifestyle tools and techniques. Often you will find that the tools and techniques that are fun to do, don't require much time, fit into your daily schedule are easy to cultivate, become a habit and will merge seamlessly into your busy life.

References

American Institute of Stress, http://stress.org/.

Bode. S, et al. (2011). Tracking the Unconscious Generation of Free Decisions." http://www.plosone.org/

Brodal, Per. *The Central Nervous System.* 4th ed. Oxford University Press, 2010.

Cannon, Walter B. *The Wisdom of the Body.* Norton.

Desikachar, T. K. V. *The Heart of Yoga.* Inner Traditions International.

Greenland, Susan K. *The Mindful Child.* Free Press, Simon and Schuster, 2010.

Ha, D. A., and S. R. George. (1989) "Neuropeptide Y-induced effects on hypothalamic corticotrophin-releasing factor" http://dx.doi.org/.

Honda's Brain Machine Interface, http://www.world.honda.com.

Human Connectome Project, http://www.humanconnectomeproject.org.

Jois, Pattabhi K. Sri. *Yoga Mala.* North Point Press.

Kataria, Madan. "Laugh For No Reason." http://www.laughteryoga.org/. Madhuri International.

Lad, Vasant. (2004) Ayurveda: The Science of Self-Healing. Lotus Press.

"Neurobiology" in *Rediscovering Biology.* http://www.learner.org/courses/biology

"Paralyzed woman uses mind to move robot arm." http://www.thejournal.el/video.

Qualcomm Tricorder X Prize. http://www.qualcommtricorderxprize.org/.

Seyle, Hans. "The Nature of Stress." http://www.icnr.com/articles/the-nature-of-stress.html.

D. J. Taylor, N. P. O. Green, and G. W. Stout. in R. Soper, ed. *Biological Science 1 & 2.* 3rd ed. Cambridge University Press.

USDA MyPlate. http://fnic.nal.usda.gov/dietary-guidance/.

VNS Therapy System-P970003s050. http://www.fda.gov/MedicalDevices/.

World Health Organization. http://www.who.int/about/definition/en/print.html.